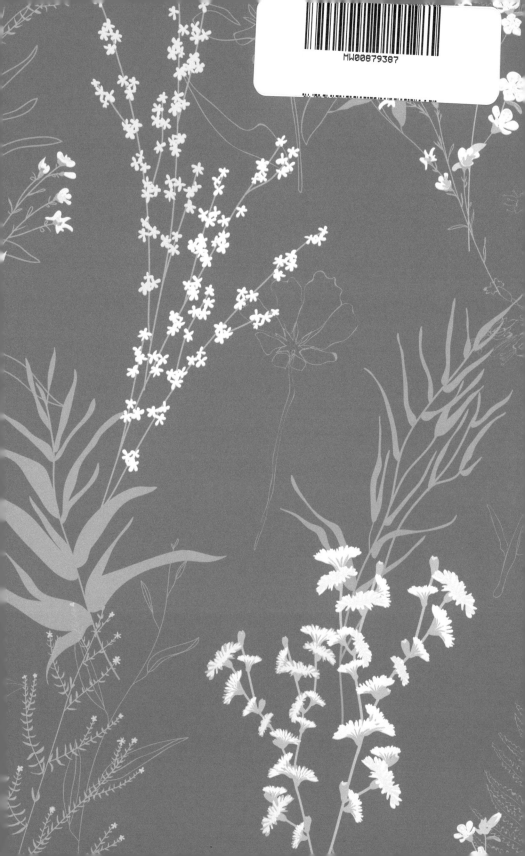

THE SOUTHERN HOME APOTHECARY
A MEDICINE GUIDE TO YOUR BACK YARD

PUBLISHED BY HIDDEN OAKS HOMESTEAD
WWW.HIDDENOAKSHOMESTEAD.COM

Disclaimer: The information presented herein is for educational purposes only and is not intended to diagnose, treat, cure, or prevent any disease. Check with your healthcare provider first if you have concerns about your health. In addition, you should speak with your healtcare provider or pharmacist before making adjustments to your diet or lifestyle and prior to introducing herbal and nutritional supplements as they may affect any treatment you may be receiving. You are advised to disclose any and all nutrient and herb supplements you are using to your healthcare team.

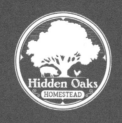

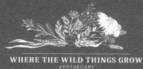

WHERE THE WILD THINGS GROW
APOTHECARY

The Southern

HOME
APOTHECARY

a medicine guide to your back yard

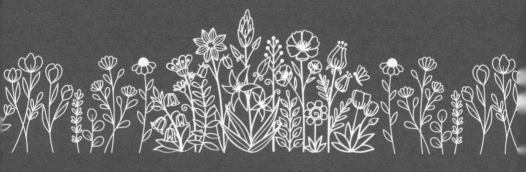

To my grandparents, who helped me discover my love for wild places, who taught me about nature's treasures and abundance. To my parents, who allowed me to be an adventure seeker in the deep forests of my childhood. To my husband, who is my biggest supporter in everything I do. To my children, who inspire me to keep ancestral knowledge alive.

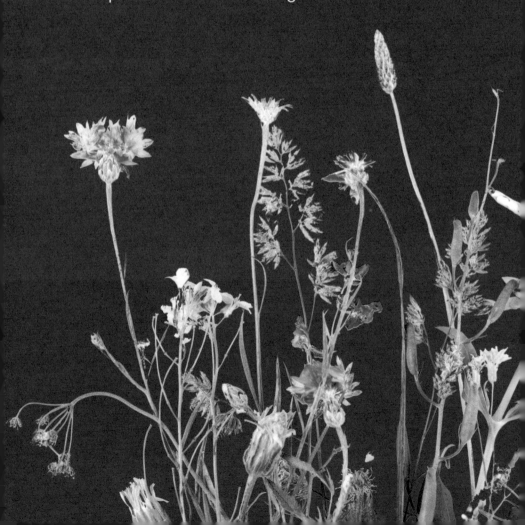

Table of CONTENTS

Hello Friends!

Through this book I am excited to share my passion for wildcrafting and foraging herbs and medicinal plants with you.

As a neighborhood herbalist, I am preserving and passing on the ancient skills that have been handed down through generations. My journey into the world of herbs began in the forests of Bavaria, where I was fortunate to learn from my grandparents, who instilled in me a deep respect and love for nature's pharmacy.

This book is a culmination of years of practice, study, and a connection to the land. It is designed to guide you through the rich tapestry of local flora, helping you identify, harvest, and utilize the incredible bounty that nature provides. Wildcrafting is more than just a method of gathering herbs; it is a way of life that fosters a deep connection with our environment and our ancestors.

In these pages, you will find information on a variety of herbs and medicinal plants, practical tips for sustainable foraging, and insights into traditional uses that have stood the test of time.

Whether you are a seasoned herbalist or a curious beginner, I hope this book will inspire you to explore the natural world with new eyes and an open heart.

By embracing these old skills, we not only enrich our own lives but also contribute to the preservation of precious ancestral knowledge.

Together, let's cultivate a deeper understanding and appreciation for the wild plants that have been our allies for countless generations.

Thank you for embarking on this journey with me. May you find joy, health, and wisdom in the practice of wildcrafting.

Nicole

First things first

What is a home apothecary?

Home apothecaries are an ancient tradition that have been passed down through many cultures for centuries. They allow you to take the healing power of plants and herbs into your own hands, and make them available for use in your daily life.

What's an herbalist?

An herbalist is someone who works with edible or medicinal plants for culinary, medicinal, or therapeutic purposes.

Herbalists study the properties of various plants and their extracts to help promote physical, mental, and emotional well being, bringing us more into balance.

Herbalists often rely on traditional knowledge and plant wisdom, but we may also incorporate modern scientific understanding of plant compounds into our practices.

Herbalists come in different shapes and forms: home, folk, community, clinical, culinary, or spiritual herbalists. There's also medicine makers, foragers, teachers, writers, aromatherapists, botanists and alchemists. All technically fall under the big "herbalist umbrella."

Starting a home apothecary is a personal journey that requires patience, curiosity, and a commitment to learning.

By taking the time to research, experiment, and cultivate your herbal knowledge, you can create a home apothecary that supports your health and well-being in a natural and holistic way.

CHAPTER 2

Foundations

WHY HERBS & PLANTS

Imagine a natural approach to wellness that involves using plants and herbs to boost your health. This method looks at your whole self – body, mind, and feelings – to help you feel your best. It's like giving your body the best plant-based support and embracing habits that keep you feeling fantastic every day.

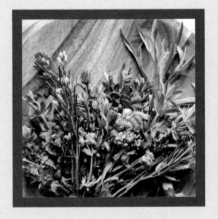

In this book we will cover easy to identify and abundant local plants, which I have personal experience with. Though there are multiple sources available covering an abundance of potential botanicals and other plants which can be found in the South East United States, this book focuses on the plants and species I have personally found, reliably identified, experimented with and made herbal applications from.

Get ready to explore the world of holistic health, where plants become your partners on the journey to a happy and healthy lifestyle!

FORAGING & WILDCRAFTING RESPONSIBLY

Foraging is an age-old practice, but it comes with a responsibility to Mother Nature. Before you set out, equip yourself with knowledge about local plant species, their seasons, and habitats. Ensure you're allowed to forage in a specific area, respecting conservation rules. Harvest modestly, leaving enough for the ecosystem to thrive. Embrace the harmony between tending to your needs and preserving the environment.

As a rule of thumb, observe the plants around you throughout the seasons. To identify plants correctly, it is important to be able to identify them during different grow, bloom and fruiting stages, as appearances can change dramatically with the seasons.

Foraging is a lifestyle choice that aligns with nature. Embrace the satisfaction of self-sufficiency, the joy of responsible foraging, and the endless possibilities of your herbal haven.

Whether you're crafting a culinary masterpiece or seeking holistic healing, start foraging, and let nature's abundance flourish in your care.

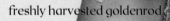

freshly harvested goldenrod

STARTING YOUR HOME APOTHECARY

Starting a home apothecary can be an exciting and rewarding journey into the world of herbal medicine and natural remedies.

Research and Education:
- Begin by educating yourself about herbal medicine, including the properties, uses, and safety considerations of different herbs.
- Invest in reputable books, online courses, or workshops on herbalism to deepen your knowledge and understanding. Even better, find a local foraging or herbalist group to get some hands-on learning done!

Identify Your Needs and Goals:
- Consider your health needs, wellness goals, and the specific conditions you want to address with herbal remedies.
- Determine whether you're interested in general wellness, first aid, managing chronic conditions, or supporting specific body systems.

Start with Basic Herbs:
- Begin by stocking your home apothecary with a selection of versatile and commonly used herbs that suit your needs and goals.
- Some essential herbs to consider for beginners include chamomile, lavender, peppermint, echinacea, and ginger.

Gather Supplies and Equipment:
- Acquire basic supplies and equipment for preparing and storing herbal remedies.
- Consider investing in tools for making herbal teas, tinctures, salves, and other preparations, such as a tea infuser, strainer, and double boiler.

Learn Basic Herbal Preparations:
- Familiarize yourself with basic methods of preparing herbal remedies, such as teas, tinctures, infusions, decoctions, salves, and poultices.
- Experiment with different preparation techniques to find what works best for you and your health needs.

Practice Safety and Caution:
- Always research the safety and contraindications of herbs before using them, especially if you have pre-existing health conditions or are pregnant or breastfeeding.
- Start with small doses and observe how your body responds to each herb, gradually increasing dosage if necessary.

Keep Records and Stay Organized:
- Maintain a journal or digital record of the herbs you use, their dosages, and the effects they have on your health.
- Label your herbal preparations with the herb name, date of preparation, and dosage instructions to ensure proper usage and avoid confusion.

Starting a home apothecary is a personal journey that requires patience, curiosity, and a commitment to learning. By taking the time to research, experiment, and cultivate your herbal knowledge, you can create a home apothecary that supports your health and well-being in a natural and holistic way.

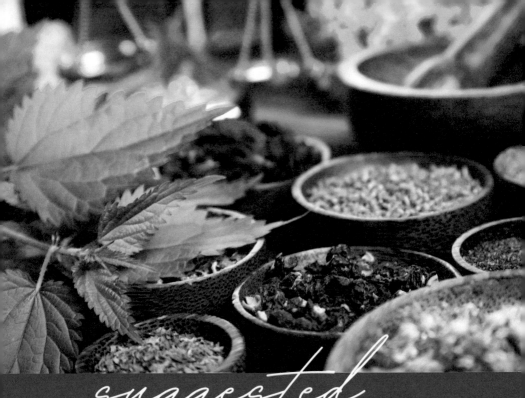

suggested
SUPPLY LIST

- glass jars
- amber bottles for storage
- mortar & pestle
- blender or coffee grinder
- sieves
- measuring cups and spoons
- bottle labels
- funnels

- 80-proof (or higher) ethyl alcohol such as vodka
- food-grade vegetable glycerin
- vinegar
- carrier oil such as olive oil
- organic bees wax

TERMINOLOGY

ELIXIR - Sweetened version of tinctures or other medicinal preparations that are created to improve the taste of extremely bitter herbs.

OXYMEL - While an oxymel is indeed an herbal elixir, not all elixirs are oxymels. The simplest definition is an herbal extraction of vinegar and raw honey. Most often, raw apple cider vinegar is used as a base, which boasts a host of healthful qualities on its own. Bringing together the acid of apple cider vinegar with the healthful properties of honey is a fantastic way to get the benefits of both, while also extracting and ingesting supportive herbs, particularly pungent ones that aren't always pleasant to take on their own.

POULTICE - a basic paste made of herbs, clays, activated charcoal, salts or other beneficial substances that is wrapped in a piece of cloth and placed on the skin.

SALVE - A salve is a mixture of fat (usually oil) and beeswax. They're usually somewhat soft, but solid at room temperature. Herbal salves are able to contain the highest concentration of herbal properties because they are such simple products and are used topically to help with wound healing, allergic reactions, and more.

SHRUB - (drinking vinegar) is a concentrated syrup that combines fruit, sugar, and vinegar. Apple cider vinegar is the most common base for shrubs, and herbs and spices are often added to create interesting flavor combinations.

SWITCHEL - another example of a delicious herbal elixir, though not necessarily sweetened with honey, Again, apple cider vinegar is the most common base used for this delicious drink. And though the preparation is the same as a shrub (as mentioned above) a switchel has the added benefits of ginger added, either as a raw herb or in a juiced version.

SYRUP - An herbal syrup is prepared by combining a concentrated decoction with either honey or sugar, and sometimes alcohol. Mixing an herbal decoction such as a glyceride or tincture, with honey or sugar helps to thicken and preserve the decoction. The basic proportions you want to use are 2 parts herbal decoction to 1 part honey or sugar. An herbal syrup, if stored correctly in a cool and dark place can be used up to 18 months.

TEA (INFUSION) - tea is the simple preparation of herbal materials by steeping them in water. This can be accomplished via hot or cold brewing your tea. While hot brewing will give you an instant product with a simple 4-6 minute steep, cold brewing will preserve more of the plant material's benefits and taste. A cold brew is accomplished by steeping the plant material 6 - 12 hours in cold water.

TINCTURE / EXTRACT - Though the process is the same, extracts are typically more potent than tinctures. In the case of extracts, the ratio of alcohol to herb is 1:1. Tinctures are made using more alcohol and less plant, with a ratio generally ranging from 3:1 to 8:1. Extracts, therefore, are administered in smaller doses than tinctures.
Both tinctures and extracts are made by covering botanical or herbal material in minimum 80 proof alcohol, and letting it sit for 4 - 6 weeks, shaking frequently. Once the tincturing process is complete, the plant material is strained out and the tincture or extract can be stored in a dark place (amber bottles are best) and used for 1-2 years.

GLYCERIDE / ALCOHOL FREE EXTRACT - the overall process to make an alcohol free tincture or extract, also called a glyceride is the same as mentioned above. The main difference lay in the fact that instead of alcohol we are using food-grade glycerine. This allows us to prepare herbal remedies for children as well as folks who cannot tolerate alcohol as a medium for the medicinal properties. The end product is typically a more syrupy consistency then an alcohol based tincture. A glyceride is typically shelf stable for up to 1 year if stored properly in a cool and dark place.

DOSING &
OTHER CONSIDERATIONS

Every herb is unique and dosages vary accordingly, but there are some general guidelines that can be very helpful.

Extract and tincture dosages can be measured in drops, dropperfuls, milliliters (mL), and teaspoons (Tsp)
- A dropperful contains about 30 drops, or 1 mL.
- 4 dropperfuls make up 3 mL, a common dosage for tinctures.
- One teaspoon (Tsp) is roughly equivalent to 5 mL.

Though there is no standardized way for dosing herbal remedies, the most commonly used dose for tinctures is 30-60 drops or 1-2 dropperfuls. In general, the more acute a condition, the more frequent the doses. Safe dosage ranges are fairly broad with most, but not all, herbs.

While many people prefer herbal medicines to some doctor-prescribed medications, others may use them in combination with prescription and nonprescription drugs.

Common uses for herbal remedies include:
- boosting the immune system
- increasing energy
- losing weight
- enhancing mood
- improving sleep

Taking herbal medicine may not be suitable for a person if they are:
- pregnant or breastfeeding
- taking prescription or OTC medications
- over age 65 and under age 18
- recent or prior surgery
- allergic to certain plant material

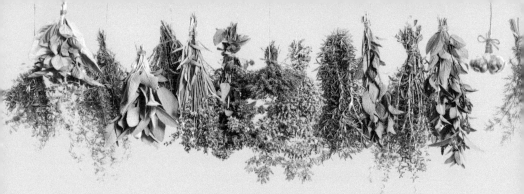

DOSING &
OTHER CONSIDERATIONS

Herbalism is a holistic health approach, based on historical data with herbal remedies which have been used for thousands of years across cultures worldwide, drawing upon the medicinal properties of various plants, roots, and botanical extracts.

Herbal medicine is usually directed towards aiding the body's own healing process. Herbal medicines usually act gently, support the body's systems and processes that have become deficient or attempt to help remove excesses that have become preponderant. Not only do herbal remedies draw from medicinal properties, they also provide diverse nutritional benefits, which in turn support the body's natural healing capacity.

Medicinal plants have been used around the world for centuries and continue to be used today; there are around 26,000 plant species with a documented medical use and some cultures rely on them heavily. In more conventional medicine, it's estimated that somewhere between 40% and 70% of all medicines in use today come from traditional or folk remedies.

Herbal treatments are steeped in traditional knowledge, much of which has been taught to the next generation through hands-on-practice. However, in recent years, through popular demand, many handbooks, workshops, group teachings and schools have spread more of this traditional knowledge.

Though supporting our bodies and health through a holistic approach is beneficial, modern medicine has it's place as well.

For any ailings, please be sure to consult with your trusted health practitioner. When basing treatments on herbal remedies, be sure to thoroughly research the plant materials you are using, and how they may affect you personally within your individual health journey.

HERBALS & COMMON AILMENTS

Digestive Issues: Beautyberry, Bidens Alba, Chickweed, Dandelion, Elder, Fleabane, Spiderwort, Wild Garlic, Honeysuckle, Magnolia, Plantain, Pine, Turkey Tail, Wood Sorrel

Insomnia and Sleep Disorders: Honeysuckle, Magnolia, Mimosa, Morning Glory, Wild Violet

Anxiety and Stress: Blackberry, Elder, Henbit, Honeysuckle, Magnolia, Mimosa, Morning Glory, Passionflower, Wild Lettuce

Brain Function: Lions Mane, Pine, Turkey Tail, Yaupon

Immune System Support: Blackberry, Brown Eyed Susan, Chickweed, Elder, Wild Garlic, Pine, Stinging Nettle, Turkey Tail, Usnea, Wood Sorrel

Pain and Inflammation: Brown Eyed Susan, Chickweed, Dandelion, Elder, Wild Garlic, Mimosa, Passionflower, Plantain, Pine, Stinging Nettle, Turkey Tail, Usnea, Wild Lettuce, Willow, Yaupon

Respiratory Issues: Brown Eyed Susan, Elder, Goldenrod, Henbit, Plantain, Pine, Red Clover, Sweet Gum, Usnea, Wild Violet

Skin Conditions: Beautyberry, Bidens Alba, Blackberry, Chickweed, Dandelion, Elder, Fleabane, Goldenrod, Plantain, Pine, Red Clover, Sweet Gum, Yaupon

Menstrual and Menopausal Symptoms: Blackberry, Fleabane, Magnolia, Morning Glory, Red Clover, Spiderwort

Urinary Tract: Dandelion, Goldenrod, Usnea, Spiderwort

Heart Health: Blackberry, Dandelion, Elder, Wild Garlic, Red Clover, Stinging Nettle

HERBAL CATEGORIES

Adaptogens:
- Adaptogens are natural substances that help the body adapt to stress and maintain balance in various physiological functions.
- They work by supporting the body's ability to cope with physical, emotional, and environmental stressors, without overstimulating or suppressing any particular system.
- Adaptogens are believed to have a normalizing effect on the body, helping to regulate hormones, improve immune function, and enhance overall well-being.
- Examples of herbal adaptogens include ashwagandha, rhodiola rosea, holy basil (Tulsi), ginseng, passionflower, morning glory, and more.

Stimulants:
- Stimulants are substances that increase physiological activity or alertness in the body, typically by stimulating the central nervous system.
- They provide a temporary boost in energy, focus, or alertness.
- Stimulants can have a rapid onset of action and may lead to feelings of euphoria, increased heart rate, elevated blood pressure, and decreased appetite.
- However, prolonged or excessive use of stimulants can lead to tolerance, dependence, and adverse health effects such as insomnia, anxiety, and cardiovascular issues.
- Examples of stimulants include caffeine (found in coffee, tea, and energy drinks) and nicotine (found in tobacco products).

While both herbal adaptogens and stimulants can affect the body's physiological responses, adaptogens primarily work to support the body's ability to adapt to stress and maintain balance, whereas stimulants provide a temporary increase in energy or alertness by stimulating the central nervous system.

Nervines: Herbs that support the nervous system, helping to calm and relax or stimulate and invigorate as needed. Examples include Honeysuckle, Magnolia, Chamomile, Lemon Balm, and Passionflower.

Diuretics: Herbs that promote urine production and increase the excretion of excess fluids from the body. Examples include Dandelion, Goldenrod, and Nettle.

Carminatives: Herbs that help relieve gas, bloating, and digestive discomfort by promoting the expulsion of gas from the digestive tract. Examples include Plantain, Fennel, and Ginger.

Astringents: Herbs that help tighten and tone tissues, useful for treating diarrhea, bleeding, and other conditions where tissue integrity needs to be restored. Examples include: Witch Hazel, Plantain, and Blackberry Leaf.

Antispasmodics: Herbs that help relieve muscle spasms and cramps by relaxing smooth muscle tissue. Examples include: Cramp Bark, Blackberry Leaves, Fleabane, and Peppermint.

While many botanicals have multiple uses and can be used inter-changeably, it is best to observe your health and body's reaction to any changes you make to your health routines.

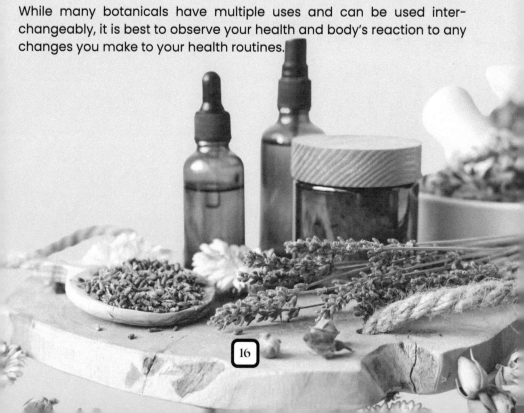

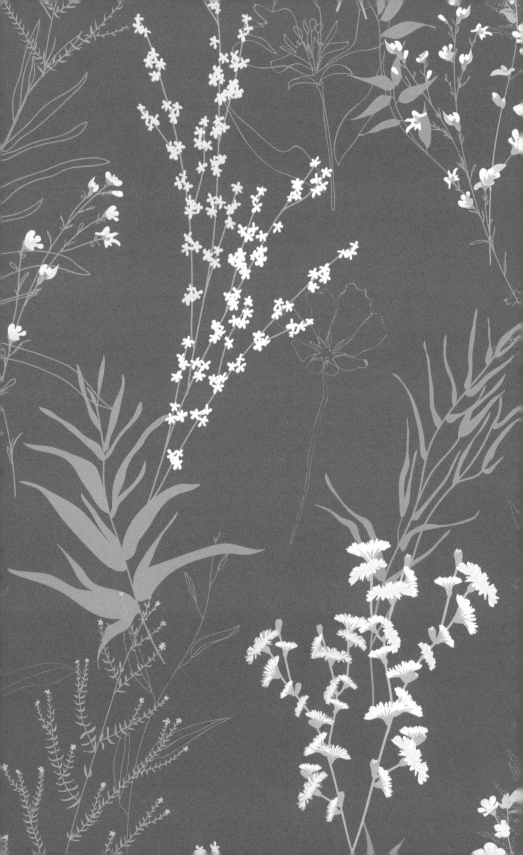

CHAPTER 3

Wild Herbs & Medicinal Plants of the Southeast US

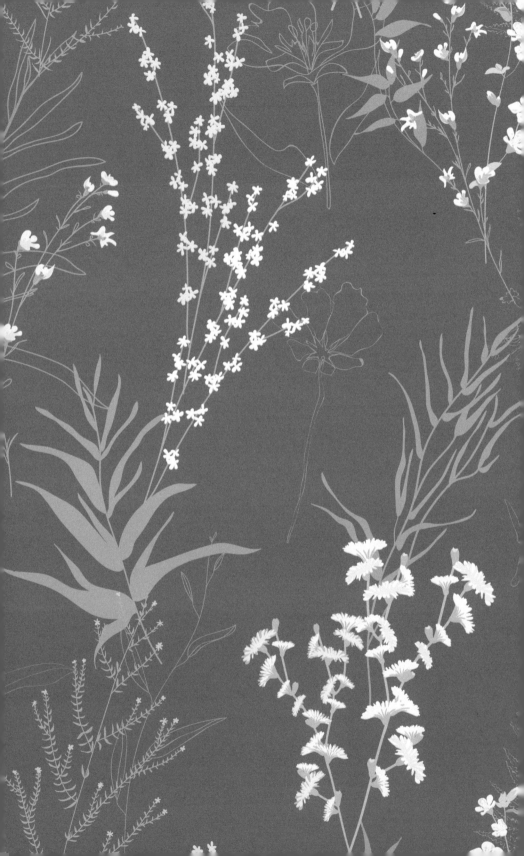

AMERICAN BEAUTYBERRY – CALLICARPA AMERICANA
BEGGARTICKS – BIDENS ALBA
BLACKBERRY – RUBUS ROSACEAE
BROWN EYED SUSAN – RUDBECKIA TRILOBA
CHICKWEED – STELLARIA MEDIA
DANDELION – TARAXACUM OFFICINALE
ELDERBERRY – SAMBUCUS NIGRA
FLEABANE – ERIGERON ANUUS
(WILD) GARLIC – ALLIUM CANADENSE
GOLDENROD – SOLIDAGO
HENBIT – LAMIUM AMPLEXICAULE
HONEYSUCKLE – LONICERA CAPRIFOLIA
LIONS'S MANE – HERICIUM ERINACEUS
(SOUTHERN) MAGNOLIA – MAGNOLIA GRANDIFLORA
MIMOSA – ALBIZIA JULIBRISSIN
MORNING GLORY – IPOMOEA INDICA
PASSION FLOWER – PASSIFLORA
(NARROWLEAF) PLANTAIN – PLANTAGO LANCEOLATA
(LONG LEAF) PINE – PINUS PALUSTRIS
POKEWEED – PHYTOLACCA DECANDRA
PRICKLY PEAR – OPUNTIA FICUS–INDICA
RED CLOVER – TRIFOLIUM PRATENSE
SPIDERWORT – TRADESCANTIA
STINGING NETTLE – UTICA DIOICA
SWEET GUM – LIQUIDAMBAR STYRACIFLUA
TURKEY TAIL – TRAMETES VERSICOLOR
USNEA – USNEA FILIPENDULA
(WILD) VIOLET – VIOLA SORORIA PRICEANA
WILD LETTUCE – LACTUA VIROSA & LACTUA SERRIOLA
(COASTALPLAIN) WILLOW – SALIX CAROLINIANA
WOOD SORREL – OXALIS
YAUPON – ILEX VOMITORIA

AMERICAN BEAUTYBERRY

Callicarpa Americana

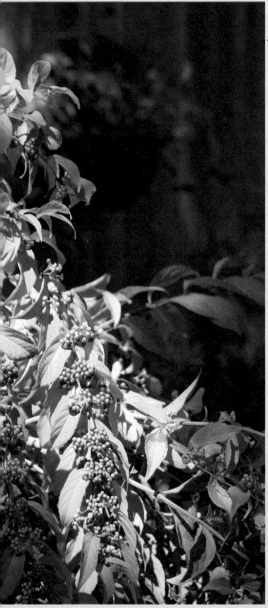

Identification

Long arching branches. Purple clusters of berries where leaves attach to stems. Leaves are oval and pointed with jagged edges. Bark: light gray-brown to gray.

Leaves have a strong citrus smell when rubbed.

When to harvest

Beautyberry blooms and forms berries in the Fall. You will usually start spotting these beautiful bright shrubs around September to October. The berries should be harvested once they turn a bright purple. I recommend harvesting in the Morning, right after the morning dew burns off.

The leaves can be harvested all year, though you will find the most tender leaves with new spring growth.

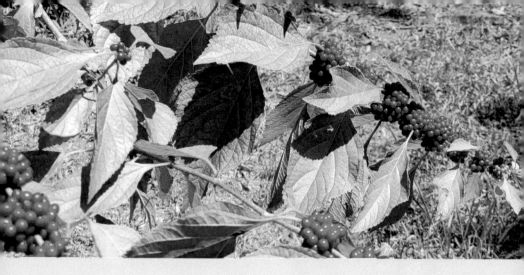

Fun Fact

Growing up, a rule of thumb we followed was: "if it's shiny and pretty, don't eat it!"

There are other beautyberry genomes, which are poisonous! In fact beautyberry plants are often used to add a splash of color to landscaping in American and European lawns and less likely to be thought of as a medicinal plant.

However, callicarpa americana is very much edible and makes a great jelly and syrup.

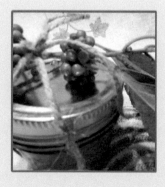

Summary

The boiled roots were made into treatments for dizziness, stomach aches, and urine retention, while bark from the stems and roots were made into concoctions for itchy skin.

Previous research found that extracts from the leaves of the beauty berry deter mosquitos and ticks. And indeed, a simple mix of water with beautyberry leaves makes a great bug-spray!

The Alabama, Choctaw, Creek, Seminole and other Native American tribes relied on the American beautyberry for various medicinal purposes. Leaves and other parts of the plant were boiled for use in sweat baths to treat malarial fevers and rheumatism.

You will spot this beautiful shrub everywhere in the South. Not only does it add a great splash of color to any late summer and fall garden, it's useful as well!

BEGGARTICKS
Bidens Alba

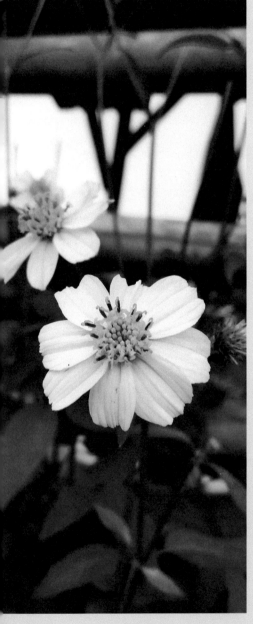

Identification

Bidens Alba has daisy-like flowers with a central disk and numerous, sharp-tipped, needle-like bracts. The leaves are toothed, and have a rough texture.

When to harvest

The plant grows to about 3-4 feet in height and blooms from late summer to early fall. Harvest depending on preferred use, whether it's the foliage or blooms you are after.

Fun Fact

Beggarticks grow at every roadside and spread easily due to the plant's ability to regrow from cut stems and the many seeds the plant produces annually.

Bidens Alba is a nutrient dense wild plant, boasting a similar nutrient profile to kale - high in fiber and proteins, carotenes, folate, and magnesium.

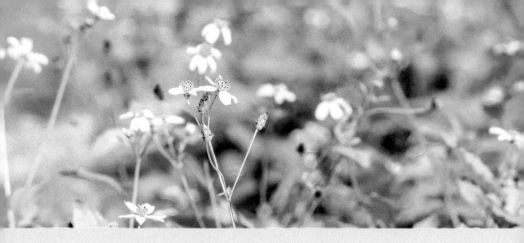

Summary

Bidens Alba has a long history of medicinal use. Many people historically and today use use leaves and flowers to treat wounds, skin diseases, and digestive problems. In traditional medicine, the plant is used as a laxative, diuretic, and to treat fever and malaria.

Some people confuse Spanish Needle with other members of the sunflower family, such as the Oxeye Daisy and the Black-Eyed Susan. It is important to be able to distinguish Bidens Alba from these look-alikes, as some of them can be toxic.

Bidens Alba is a versatile plant that many people use for medicinal and culinary purposes. Whether used as a tea or as a seasoning, this plant is a valuable resource for botanists and herbalists alike.

People in South Africa, Zulus, and the people of India consume the fresh or dried leaves by boiling them. Young leaves of this plant may also be eaten as a salad.

Bidens alba contains saponins, so older leaves may be unpleasant to the taste and may upset your stomach.

BLACKBERRY
Rubus Rosaceae

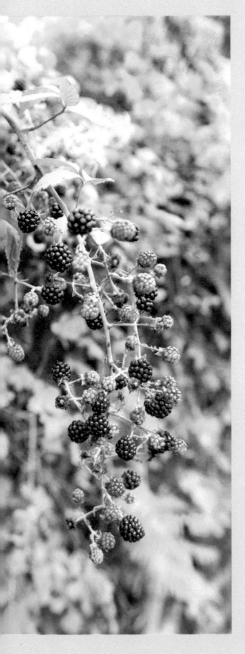

Identification

Blackberry plants have biennial canes (stems) that are characteristically covered with prickles and are erect, semi-erect, or trailing. The compound leaves usually feature three or five oval, coarsely toothed, stalked leaflets, many of which persist through the winter. The flowers are white, pink, or red and produce black or red-purple fruits.

When to harvest

The stems can easily grow 8 - 10 feet. Flowers will appear in spring, followed by the berries, which will be ready to harvest early summer. Leaves can be harvested year-round, though the most tender growth will be in the Spring.

Fun Fact

Blackberry, Raspberry, Dewberry, etc. are in the same plant family as roses. Surprised?

Though commonly called berries, the fruits of Rubus species are technically aggregates of drupelets. The drupelets of blackberries remain attached to a juicy white core.

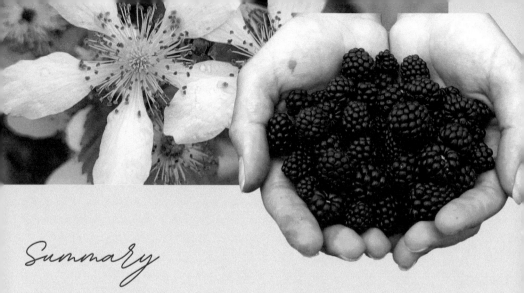

Summary

Blackberries are a fairly good source of iron, vitamin C, and antioxidants and are generally eaten fresh, in preserves, or in baked goods such as cobblers and pies.

Even the leaves have a long history of use for its healthful properties. Blackberry leaves can be used as a gentle astringent tonic in herbal teas and have a pleasant, fruity flavor. Blackberry leaf can also be applied in topical applications such as toners, washes, lotions, and more.

Blackberries are packed with vitamins, minerals, fiber and antioxidants. Research studies show that antioxidants may reduce inflammation and prevent many diseases. The nutrients in blackberries improve digestion and blood sugar levels.

One of blackberries' main claims to fame is that they're bursting with strong antioxidants called polyphenols. Antioxidants help you fight stress by destroying unstable molecules called free radicals before they can damage your cells.

Blackberries may also help with cardiovascular disease and conditions that affect your heart and blood vessels. A common cause of cardiovascular disease is when plaque builds up inside of your arteries.

Nutrients in blackberries also improve brain function through increasing blood flow to your brain and activating areas that control speech, memory and attention. They can also improve speech and memory in people with mild or moderate dementia.

BROWN-EYED SUSAN

Rudbeckia Triloba

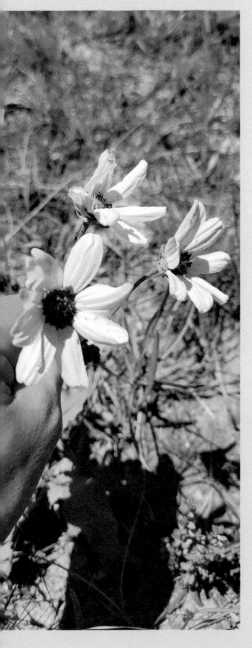

Identification

Upright flowering plant that can be either biennial or perennial depending on the climate it is found in. This herb belongs to the sunflower (coneflower) family or the family Asteraceae.

It is a popular garden plant but is also found growing wild in fields and along roadsides. It can reach 2 to 3 feet in height.

The leaves are alternate and mostly basal covered by rather coarse hairs.

When to harvest

The Brown-eyed Susan is a widely spread wildflower, blooming during spring and sometimes again during fall. You can find it on roadsides and ditches all over the Southeast United States. I do not recommend foraging from roadsides ever, due to pollution. Harvesting should be done at a distance of a minimum 30 feet from any roadside.

Fun Fact

There are no reports of side effects associated with the use of Brown-eyed Susan root. However, the seeds are not recommended for human consumption.

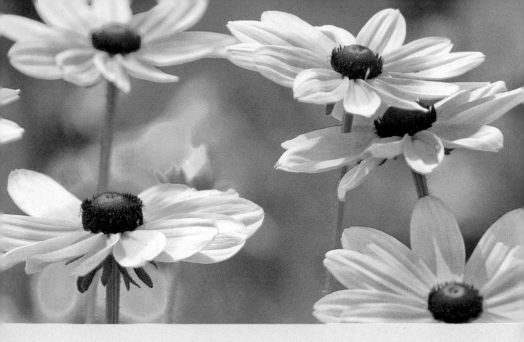

Summary

The Brown-eyed Susan has a long history of use in traditional medicine. The plant has been used to treat various ailments, including respiratory problems, fever, and sore throat. The plant is known to have anti-inflammatory properties, which makes it useful in treating respiratory issues such as bronchitis, asthma, and chest congestion.

This common wildflower has been used for centuries as a medicinal herb by various native North American tribes to treat a wide range of ailments and even if it is not one of the most recognized medicinal plants it still has its uses in modern herbal medicine.

Recent studies indicate that extracts made from the brown-eyed Susan root can be beneficial in stimulating the immune system and in that regard being even more effective than the better known Echinacea. They are, after all, part of the same plant family and therefore have similar immune boosting properties.

The root has been used traditionally as an herbal remedy to rid the body of parasitic worms. The Ojibwa also made a poultice or external wash made from this herb as a treatment for snake bites.

CHICKWEED | STITCHWORT

Stellaria Media

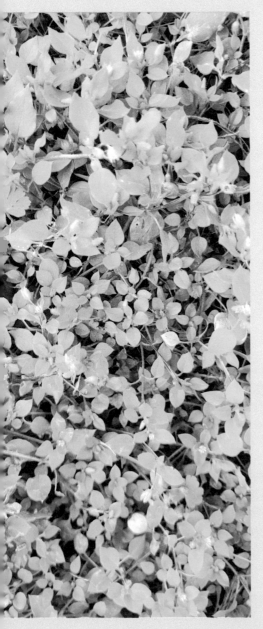

Identification

Species of chickweed have inconspicuous but delicate, white, somewhat star-shaped flowers.

The common chickweed is native to Europe but is widely naturalized. It usually grows to 18 inches but becomes a low-growing and spreading annual weed in mowed lawns.

It likes cooler climates, which for the SE US means, it tends to be a winter perennial. Our weather usually turns too hot and humid by early April.

When to harvest

Chickweed is a readily available perennial which will pop up in lawns, gardens, freshly disturbed areas and everywhere else every spring.

Chickweed typically starts showing up once day temperatures reach 50F. However it likes cooler temperatures and will start dying back quickly once day temperatures reach 75F and higher.

This plant is extremely prolific and will spread easily, which makes it an amazing wild plant to harvest to your heart's desire.

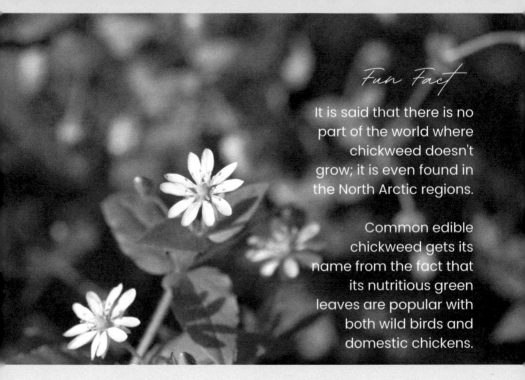

Summary

Chickweed is abundant in lawns, sidewalks, and open areas. Stellaria media has been a useful and beneficial herb in traditional European healing practices for centuries. The fresh leaves can be eaten raw in salads, and dried chickweed herb is often infused as chickweed tea, macerated in vinegars, tinctured, or used in skin care creations.

Chickweed is a fast-growing plant that has been utilized as a folk remedy for many conditions, including arthritis pains, skin conditions, such as rashes and eczema, asthma, constipation, and kidney related issues.

Chickweed is safe to eat and is high in antioxidants, saponins, vitamins C and A, and a number of other anti-inflammatory compounds. You can eat it both raw or cooked, and unlike some other nutrient-dense plants, such as dandelion or mustard greens for example, chickweed is described as having a pleasant and mild taste that is not very bitter. Its taste is closer to spinach, in my opinion.

As medicinal, whether consumed as a tea, tincture of fresh juice, or applied to the skin as a compress or salve, chickweed can be used to help decrease swelling, pain, redness and congestion.

DANDELION

Taraxacum Officinale

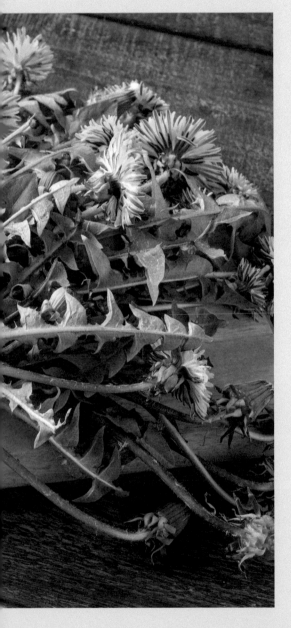

Identification

The dandelion is a readily identifiable, hardy, perennial weed. It has a rosette base producing several flowering stems and multiple leaves.

Dandelions have toothy, deeply-notched, basal leaves that are hairless. They are 2 to 10 inches or longer and they form a rosette above the central taproot.

When to harvest

Dandelion is a spring plant and will return each year if you will allow it to go to seed. You can harvest the flower heads once they are fully opened and right after the morning dew dries up.

Leaves get more bitter with maturity of the plant, making young leaves the best for salads. The root can be harvested once the plant reaches full maturity.

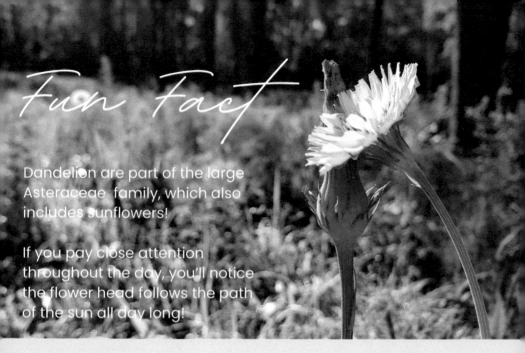

Fun Fact

Dandelion are part of the large Asteraceae family, which also includes Sunflowers!

If you pay close attention throughout the day, you'll notice the flower head follows the path of the sun all day long!

Summary

Dandelions are often considered a pesky weed, yet growing up in Europe, I have greatly benefited for years from the incredible nutritional value that this weed contains. They are a rich source of vitamins, minerals and it even has antioxidants. For example, one cup of raw dandelion greens contains 112% of your daily required intake of vitamin A and 535% of vitamin K. The common yellow dandelion has a long list of powerful healing abilities as well as other health benefits. Contrary to popular belief, this is a beneficial plant to have.

It's a great companion plant for gardening because its long taproot brings up nutrients to shallow-rooting plants in the garden adding minerals and nitrogen to the soil. It also attracts pollinating insects.

Dandelions are also often found in herbal teas and supplements, where they're used as a natural remedy to support blood sugar management and boost skin, liver, and heart health.

From root to flower, dandelions are highly nutritious plants loaded with vitamins, minerals, and fiber. Dandelions contain high levels of the antioxidant beta-carotene, which protects against cell damage and oxidative stress, and therefore chronic disease.

Dandelion contains bioactive compounds that have been shown to reduce blood sugar, may protect against liver damage, and due to it's high fiber content and prebiotic compounds supports healthy digestion. It's a natural and abundant super food!

ELDERBERRY

Sambucus Nigra

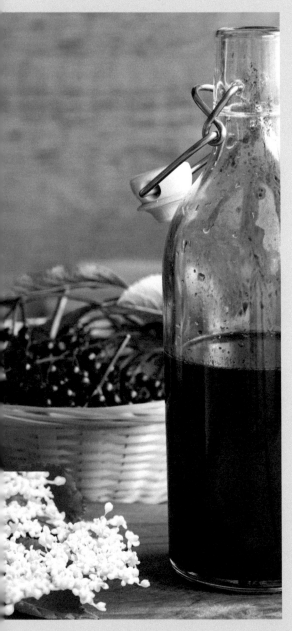

Identification

If you want to identify an elderberry plant in your area, look for clusters of small white flowers, drooping purple fruit, and hard, woody bark.

When identifying plants, I recommend to observe over the seasons for the best and most reliable identification.

Never eat the seeds, stems, leaves, or roots of the elderberry plant, as they are toxic in high doses.

When to harvest

Elder grows as a perennial shrub. Flower heads can be harvested in late spring. The berries will usually ripen up towards the end of summer, if you are able to beat the birds and other wildlife to them.

Fun Fact

Did you know the flower make a delicious treat?

In fact, in Europe the flower of the elder plant is used just as often as the berry, and makes great syrup, fritters, cordials, and more...

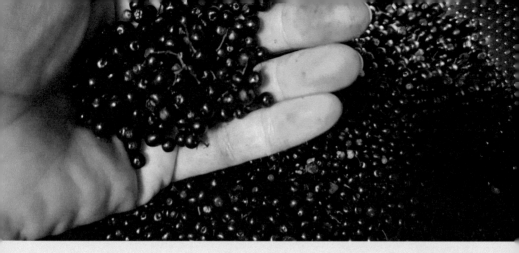

Summary

In folk medicine, the dried berries or juice are used to treat influenza, infections, sciatica, headaches, dental pain, heart pain, and nerve pain, as well as a laxative and diuretic. Additionally the berries can be cooked and used to make juice, jams, chutneys, pies and elderberry wine.

The berries and flowers of elder are packed with antioxidants and vitamins that boost your immune system. They help tame inflammation, lessen stress, and help protect your heart, too.

Elderberry juice is also linked to weight loss, reduced blood pressure, and improved well-being.

Elder grows as a shrub, and is prolific in most growing zones. It does well in drainage ditches, where it is often found. Elderberry shrubs do really well under both flood and drought conditions.

They are an excellent plant to try out your plant multiplication skills, as they are extremely easy to harvest cuttings from and subsequently root. Elders are also very forgiving to weather conditions and do well even in very poor soil, as well as in drought or flood conditions, once established.

FLEABANE

Erigeron Annuus

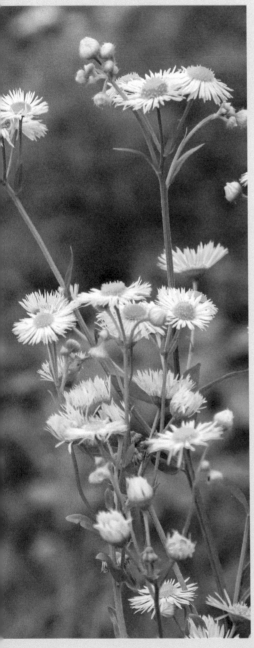

Identification

It typically blooms late spring and forms fuzzy white seed heads while still producing new flowers.

It's one of the many medicinal wildflowers within the Asteraceae family, which also includes cone flowers in all shapes and forms, dandelions and sunflowers.

When to harvest

As their scientific name indicates fleabane is an annual wildflower and can be temperamental. This beautiful flower may be in abundance one year, and then hard to find the next year. It all depends on the level of seed germination each year.
When harvesting, leave enough flower heads for them to go to seed and return the next year.

Fun Fact

Fleabane has been used as an insect repellant in folklore all over the world, from Europe to America.
Old stories tell of the weed being used in animal beddings and also human sleeping quarters where bunches of the plant were hung at the foot of the bed to keep bed bugs away.

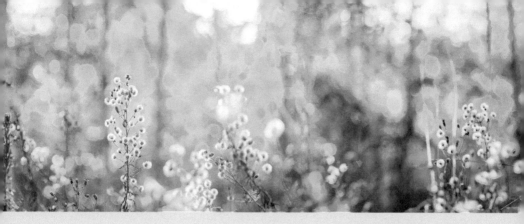

Summary

Though common fleabane is in the same plant family as dandelion, echinacea, and brown-eyed susans, much less of the actual plant is usable. With fleabane, only the leaves are edible. They are hairy so they have a somewhat 'furry' texture making eating them raw not exactly pleasing. They can be used wherever you cook with greens.

Daisy fleabane leaf extracts contain caffeic acid which is an active compound that has antioxidative and neuroprotective effects and therefore is an excellent medium to protecting our brain cells.

Fleabane is primarily said to support the digesting, integumentary and reproductive systems, therefore the uses typically concentrate on supporting skin and digestive issues.

Common usage includes tea brewed from the roots to help stimulate and normalize menstrual flow. Hence, do not ingest if pregnant or trying to conceive.

Of course, there is also the typical astringent uses of the leaves and flowers in forms of poultices for sores and as a diuretic for kidney stones.

(WILD) GARLIC

Allium Canadense

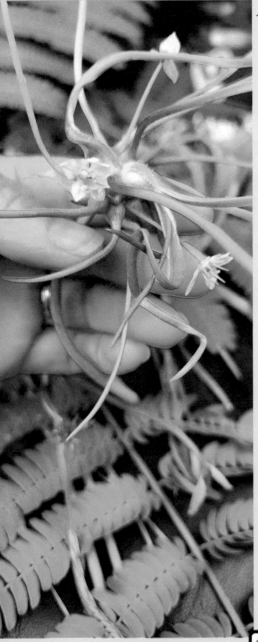

Identification

The wild garlic plant is a medium-sized bulbous perennial which can grow up to 2 feet height.

It has a distinctive and pungent garlicky smell that perfumes woodlands in spring. The flowers are small, white, with six petals and can be found on the end of a thin stalk.

When to harvest

Wild garlic is best harvested in the spring, when the leaves are vibrant green and before the plants bloom.

Look for young plants in shady, damp areas where they thrive. They should be picked carefully without uprooting the entire plant, which is crucial to preserving the wild population.

For fresh harvesting target the leaves from close to the base and snip them with scissors.

In general, bulb harvesting should be avoided to prevent disrupting the plant's ability to regrow

Fun Fact

The simplest tip to help identify wild garlic is the smell.

The leaves of poisonous look alikes like lily-of-the-valley do not smell of garlic at all. The same tip applies to the flowers, lily-of-the-valley smells sweet and, well.. flowery.

Smell as you forage to help identify wild garlic, but if you are on a woodland walk it can also help you to find a hidden patch, if you pay attention.

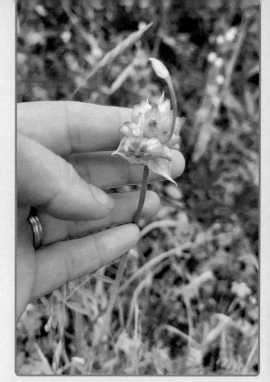

Summary

From its antioxidant and anti-inflammatory properties to its ability to aid cardiovascular health by reducing blood clotting and lowering cholesterol levels, this versatile plant offers a myriad of benefits.

Sulphur compounds in the plant act as antioxidants, protecting the body from free radicals and preventing degenerative diseases. These compounds also possess anti-inflammatory properties, aiding in fighting infections and reducing inflammation in the body.

This amazing wild food can slightly reduce blood clotting. It can also help lower blood cholesterol levels, reduce blood pressure, and help prevent strokes and other cardiovascular issues.

Wild garlic, just like it's cousins, has antibacterial, antimicrobial, antibiotic, antiseptic, and antiparasitic effects, helping the body fight infections and kill parasites. It's also a great help with digestive ailments and can protect from stomach ulcers and benefit the gut wall and gut health in general.

GOLDENROD

Solidago

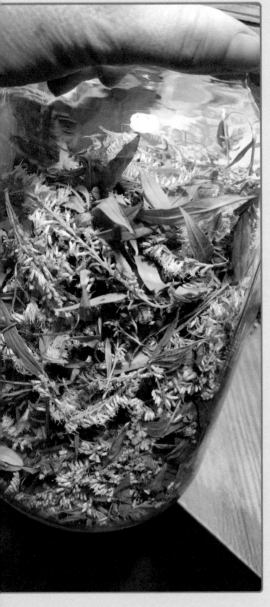

Identification

Goldenrod grows in many different growing zones, ranging from zones 2 to 10 in different shapes and forms.

In the Southeast United States it blooms in fall and is easily identified by it's bright yellow blooming "rods."

When to harvest

Goldenrod tends to be pretty prolific, though continued de-forestation and development is taking away large wild fields of this amazing plant.

Goldenrod blooms in the fall. The flowers and leaves can be harvested before the flowers appear and used directly. It's best to harvest flowers right before they reach full bloom.

Fun Fact

Goldenrod is often blamed for seasonal allergies.

However, Ragweed, which blooms the same time of year, is the real troublemaker. Goldenrod will actually alleviate allergy symptoms.

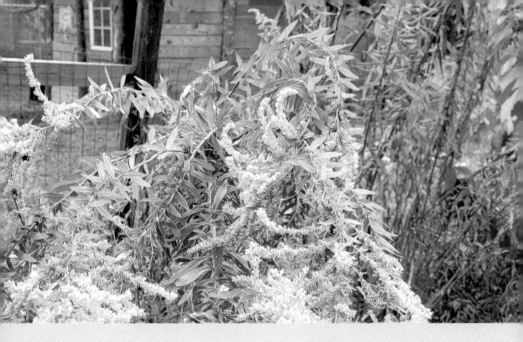

Summary

Goldenrod is a premier decongestant, effectively alleviating upper respiratory congestion stemming from allergies, sinusitis, flu, or the common cold. It can be taken as a tea, syrup, or tincture for this purpose.

Goldenrod also has an affinity for the urinary tract and is used as a diuretic, antimicrobial, and anti-inflammatory as a remedy for urinary tract infections. The diuretic quality of goldenrod may also help to relieve edema, gout, and kidney stones.

Goldenrod's piney tasting leaves and flowers are an important medicinal remedy for the urinary, digestive, and respiratory system. The goldenrod genus encompasses one hundred species of late-blooming, knee- or hip high herbaceous perennials.

Much of what we know about goldenrod's medicinal uses comes from folk and native wisdom, where various goldenrod species are traditionally used for a number of ailments, both topically and internally.

Topically goldenrod is an important dermatological aid for sores, infections, toothaches, burns, and wounds.

HENBIT
Lamium Amplexicaule

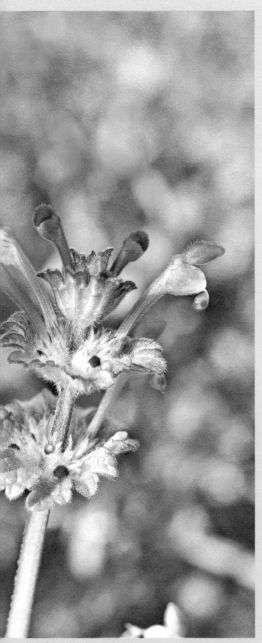

Identification

Henbit is a low-growing annual plant growing 4-10 inches tall, with soft, finely hairy stems.
The leaves are opposite, rounded, about 1 inch in diameter.
The flowers are pink to purple. The specific name refers to the amplexicaul leaves (leaves grasping the stem.)

When to harvest

Henbit is another spring blooming plant and one of the first blooms our bees will visit coming out of winter hibernation. The entire plant is edible and usable, however, the leaves and stems get woody as they mature, so younger plants and leaves make a more tender salad.

Fun Fact

Henbit has a bad reputation as an invasive weed. Did you know it's rich in Vitamins A, C, E, and K and it boosts Iron and Magnesium, too?

It makes a beautiful salve and tincture, but is great fresh in a salad or as a tea, as well.

Though it's in the mint family, it tastes nothing like it. In fact, it's pretty pleasant, with a sweet, peppery taste.

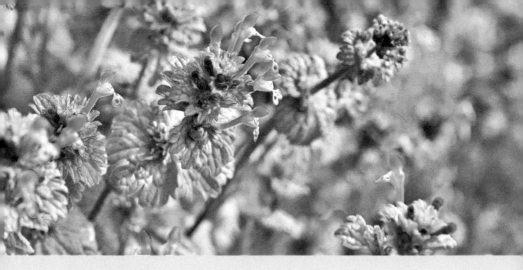

Summary

I discovered henbit, true to it's title as a weed, making itself comfortable everywhere in my garden. Inside my raised beds, in the walkways, in little crevices, everywhere.

True to my nature, I did some research and found it is edible, which prompted me to add it to my salad the same day. I quite like the taste of it, and the little hairy stems did not bother me one bit.

After a bit more research, I found out that all above-ground parts of henbit – the stems, flowers, and leaves – are edible. But, like other early spring plants, the stems get tougher as they mature. So, you might want to stick to younger plants. Depending on who you ask, some may say henbit tastes almost like raw kale or celery. This plant doesn't have a strong aroma, just a pleasant and mild earthy smell with a light minty note on top.

Low in calories and rich in vitamins, minerals, and fiber, henbit is a great ingredient to add to your diet. It also has some amazing natural medicinal qualities. Henbit has been used in herbal remedies to reduce fever, induce sweating, and treat joint aches.

Some people create henbit green smoothies to aid digestion and boost energy. And henbit herbal tea has stimulant and excitant effects which means it could help relieve stress and anxiety.

While henbit is a fantastic food to forage, overeating the leaves or drinking too much henbit tea could produce a laxative effect.

HONEYSUCKLE

Lonicera Caprifolia

Identification

Honeysuckle plants can be evergreen or deciduous, with simple leaves arranged oppositely along the stems.

The winter leaf buds have distinctive scales. Most species have two-lipped fragrant flowers with a sweet nectar. The tubular flowers are commonly borne in pairs.

The fruit is a red, orange, or black berry that is attractive to wildlife.

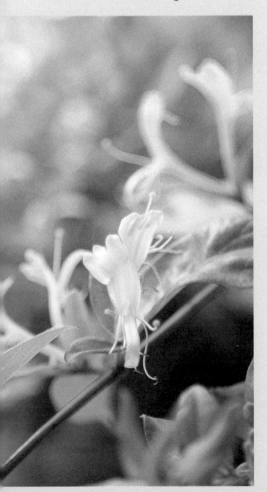

When to harvest

Honeysuckle is another spring forage and bloom. Remember to share it's goodness with your pollinators.

Fun Fact

Eating or sucking honeysuckle as a kid probably triggers some happy memories for some, though I did not discover this plant until I moved to our land in Florida.

Though all honeysuckle species flowers are edible and our local honeysuckle is usually safe, it's important to identify plants correctly. The berries of the Dwarf Honeysuckle (Fly Honeysuckle) and Tartarian Honeysuckle are toxic.

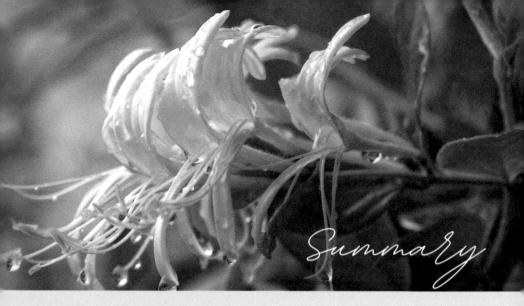

The flowers, seeds, berries, and leaves have been used for medicine for hundreds of years. Honeysuckle is commonly used for indigestion, bacterial or viral infections, to increase memory, treat diabetes, the common cold, and many other conditions. As with many herbal remedies and medicinal uses, scientific evidence is scarce and the knowledge of the plants and their properties is in many cases handed down from generation to generation.

Honeysuckle makes an excellent natural remedy for removing heat from the body as well as toxins. Traditional Chinese Medicine practitioners use the flower both internally and externally for a variety of health conditions including skin infections, ulcers, fevers and inflammatory conditions.

Native Americans were known to boil the fresh honeysuckle leaves with water to use on wounds to encourage healing. There are quite a few benefits to using honeysuckle for natural healing, including its ability to manage blood sugar levels, treat symptoms of nausea, and reduce inflammation throughout the body, among others.

You can apply a tincture of infusion to boils to reduce their size and treat the pain. Honeysuckle tea can eliminate inflammation in the respiratory tracts associated with bronchitis and sore throat.

In aromatherapy, honeysuckle can help in relaxation and sinus pressure relief, among others. The fragrance of honeysuckle is often also used in it's essential oil form in perfumes and other fragrant applications.

LION'S MANE MUSHROOM

Hericium Erinaceus

Identification

Lion's mane mushroom is a shaggy white orb suspended boldly against a landscape of rich red and yellow autumn hues. Specimens can grow over a foot across, though many remain a more modest seven to ten inches. Lion's Mane rarely reaches peak prime at only two or three inches.

- White fruiting body
- Long hair-like or tooth-like spines
- Growing in fall or winter
- Growing on hardwood
- Sweet scent
- Growing on deadwood, sick wood, or tree wounds

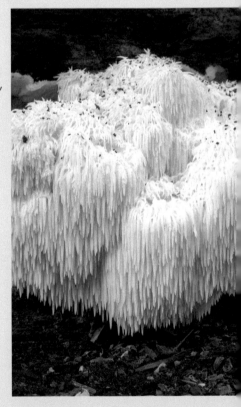

When to harvest

Early spring and summer are the best time to harvest this amazing fungi wild. If you are looking for a reliable supply, lion's mane is extremely easy to grow at home in order to have fresh supply all year round.

Fun Fact

This species goes by 'bearded tooth mushroom,' 'pom pom mushroom,' 'monkey head mushroom', and 'yamabushitake,' a Japanese word that translates to "those who sleep in the mountains."

This specific fungi can easily be grown from mushroom grow kits.

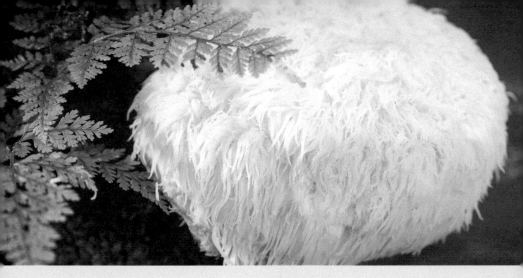

Summary

I have yet harvested a wild one, and the last large one I ran into was hauled away with a timber truck as it was growing on a cut down pine tree. So I keep my eyes open when I am foraging as I know they do indeed grow well in the Southeast. I wanted to include this amazing fungi due to it's many benefits and the fact that they can be easily identified and found wild here.

Lion's mane is edible and delicious fried in butter, but it's even better as a medicinal mushroom. It can be tinctured or dehydrated and powdered and therefore added to foods of all kind to add nutrition and health benefits to any dish. Lately it has become popular to grind up mushrooms and add them to coffee, make a hot chocolate mix or add them to teas and smoothies.

Lion's Mane is known for it's support of brain function and brain health, including it's support in treating anxiety, depression and chronic inflammation.

In addition, the properties found in this wonderful mushroom also support heart health, gut health, the digestive system, and is an overall immune booster.

(SOUTHERN) MAGNOLIA

Magnolia Grandiflora

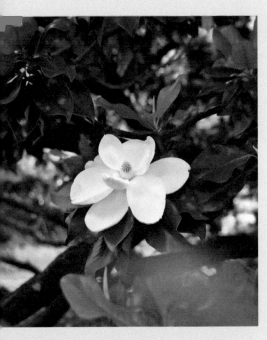

Identification

The Southern Magnolia is an evergreen tree and maintains her dark green, glossy leaves throughout the year.

Though it's wise to observe through the season, the large glossy, leathery leaves help to easily identify even new growth trees before they are ever large or old enough to carry their beautiful blooms.

When to harvest

Magnolias bloom in spring and summer. Once flowers start to come to maturity, they are ready to be harvested for teas. However, the flower buds also make an excellent foraged food. Since this beautiful tree is an evergreen in our parts, the leaves can be harvested all year long, though young growth is most tender.

!WARNING!

Magnolia extracts and supplements are extremely powerful and is not recommended in large doses.
Moreover, magnolia supplements shouldn't be used by pregnant women, as they are known to cause vertigo, dizziness, and headaches.
Its bark contains high concentrations of chemicals and can cause respiratory paralysis in animals or infant children.

Fun Fact

Magnolia trees are ancient, with a history dating back over 95 million years, making them one of the oldest flowering plants on Earth.
These majestic trees have witnessed the rise and fall of various civilizations and have remained a symbol of strength and endurance throughout the ages.

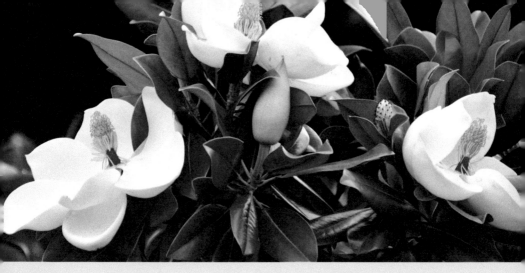

Summary

Both the bark and flower buds can be used to make medicine. Magnolia is used for weight loss, problems with digestion, constipation, inflammation, anxiety, stress, depression, fever, headache, stroke, and asthma. The flower bud is used for stuffy nose, runny nose, common cold, sinus pain, hay fever, headache, and facial dark spots. There's a multitude of uses for this tree, besides the fact that it attracts pollinators, and adds beauty to any landscape.

By regulating the endocrine system, magnolia might help reduce anxiety and stress by soothing the mind and lowering hormone release in the body. A similar chemical pathway allows it to help relieve depression as well.

Components found in magnolia flowers and bark are also considered soothing or relaxing agents, reducing inflammation and muscle tension when consumed. Magnolia supplements are often recommended, as they may provide relief for menstrual cramps, as well as improve mood.

If you have hay fever, seasonal allergies, or specific allergen sensitivity, magnolia supplements can help strengthen your resistance and keep you feeling your best!

Magnolia bark's active compounds mimics cortisol and has the potential to help the body control its release and management of blood sugar.

Along with stimulating the lymphatic system and increasing the level of toxins being eliminated from the body, magnolia has also been linked to reducing the build-up of fat around the liver.

Magnolia Seed Pod

MIMOSA TREE
(PERSIAN SILK TREE | HAPPINESS TREE)
Albizia Julibrissin

Identification

The Persian Silk Tree is a fast-growing, short-lived, small to medium size deciduous tree. It typically is found along roadsides, grasslands, vacant lots, clearings, or flood plain areas and is considered an invasive species.

The tree has a broad crown and may have single or multiple trunks. Its height typically ranges from 10-50 feet and its spread is 20-50 feet.

Observing over the seasons can help to identify this tree easily when in bloom.

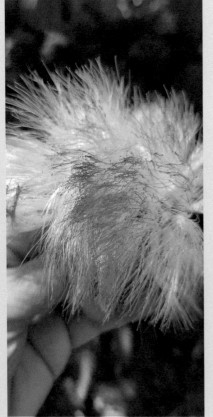

When to harvest

Mimosa blooms early summer, and you will be able to smell the heavenly scent heavy in the air surrounding the tree.

Pollinators absolutely love this tree. The flower buds can be harvested and used fresh, or used dried or tinctured. Besides the flowers, the bark can be harvested for it's medicinal properties.

Fun Fact

The mimosa tree is native to Asia and the Middle East and was imported to the US as an ornamental tree. Due to it's beautiful blooms and attracting pollinators with it's nectar and smell it made a great, colorful addition in landscaping.

Due to its medicinal properties in supporting mental health, it has been dubbed as the "Happiness Tree".

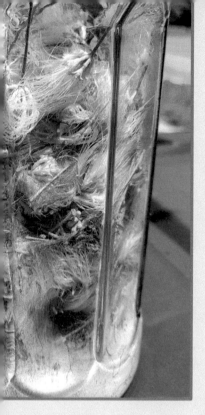

Summary

All parts of the mimosa tree have been used for medicine, sustenance, and material, cross-culturally and throughout millennia.

Mimosa tree bark and flowers have been traditionally used in herbal medicine to alleviate anxiety and stress-related symptoms. The tree contains compounds such as alkaloids, flavonoids, and saponins that have sedative properties, helping to calm the mind and promote relaxation.

The Mimosa tree is renowned for its mood-enhancing effects. The leaves and flowers are often prepared as infusions or tinctures, believed to uplift the spirit and improve overall well-being. These preparations may help combat feelings of sadness, melancholy, and promote a sense of positivity.

In certain traditional practices, the Mimosa tree has been utilized as a natural remedy for insomnia. Its calming properties can help soothe the nervous system, facilitating a more restful sleep and promoting a refreshed awakening.

The bark and leaves of the Mimosa tree contain compounds with anti-inflammatory and antioxidant properties. These attributes may contribute to reducing inflammation in the body.

MORNING GLORY

Ipomoea Indica

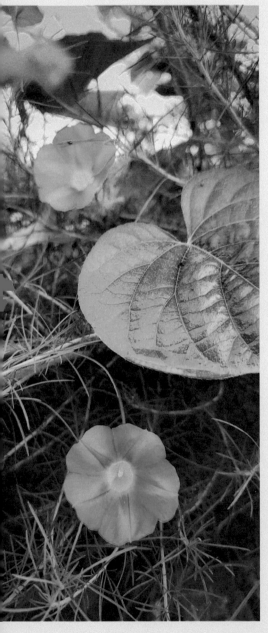

Identification

Morning Glory comes in many different colors and shapes. However our native type has a light blue flower and heart shaped leaves, similar to sweet potato and wild potato vines.

When to harvest

This plant is incredibly prolific and will return each year. If not managed, it can easily spread and get invasive. The entire plant is edible, though the flowers and seeds come with medicinal properties.

Flowers should be harvested after morning dew to assure the highest concentration of oils. Leaves and vines can be harvested at any time during blooming season, which lasts from spring into summer and fall.

Fun Fact

Morning glory has deep symbolic meaning in various cultures. It is often associated with love, affection, and emotional bonds. In Chinese folklore, morning glory represents the pursuit of love and the journey of the soul. In Victorian flower language, morning glory symbolizes love, affection, and a deep connection with a loved one.

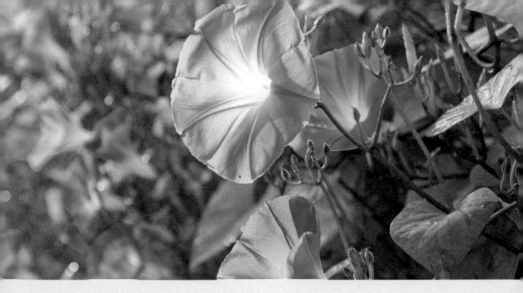

Summary

The flower is noted to have remarkably purifying, calming, and cleansing effects which scientists believe indicate the plant's anti-inflammatory and antioxidant compounds.

The flower is used therapeutically to combat the effects of stress. Morning glories make people feel calm and peaceful.

Morning glory is believed to have antibacterial and antifungal properties. Chinese herbalists also recommend the plant as an anti-diabetic medication. They believe that the plant keeps blood sugar levels in check.

Native Americans used to crush the flower and apply it topically as an antidote for spider bites.

The plant can be considered an adaptogen, although it's more potent as a calming agent. Some research has shown promise in lowering the heart rate and lessening the negative effects caused by stress and worry. Morning glories play a specific role as to how the brain responds to external stimuli and can support cognitive function.

!WARNING!

A word of caution, though: Morning Glory has the same toxicological profile as many tranquilizers and antipsychotic medications.

They should not be taken alongside some other prescriptive medicine or alternative healing roots for depression such as St. John's Wort.

PASSION FLOWER MAYPOP

Passiflora

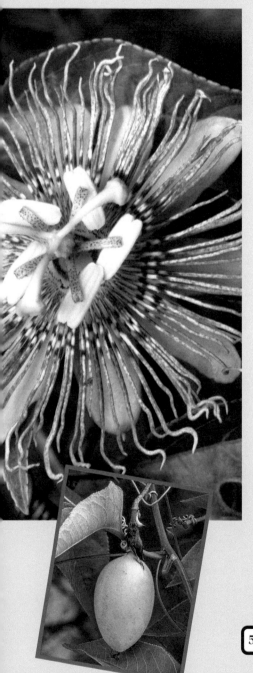

Identification

A passionflower has a wide, flat petal base with five or 10 petals in a flat or reflex circle. Passionflowers are rapid growers, coming back every year in zones 7-11.

The wild passion flower can climb about 10 to 30 feet high and has flowers ranging from white, through pink and purple. As the plant matures it produces a yellow berrylike edible fruit about 2-3 inches in size.

When to harvest

This is an extremely prolific plant, though, if not cultivated, it could take a bit to find and locate good vines.

The blooms are usually showing off in late summer and early fall.. However, since all of the plant is usable, in our region it can be harvested all year for leaves.

The fruit is edible and makes a delightful treat.

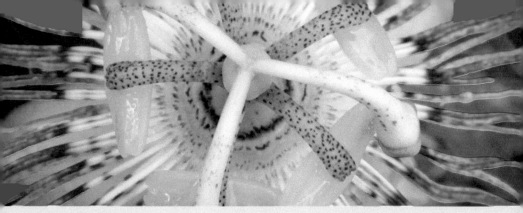

Fun Fact

Early Christian missionaries decided to capitalize on its distinctive morphology, and use it as an educational tool in describing Christ's crucifixion. The name describes the passion of Christ and his disciples.

Summary

Passionflower is a valuable sedative and tranquillising herb with a long history of use in North America. It is frequently used in the treatment of insomnia, epilepsy, and hysteria. The leaves and stems are antispasmodic, astringent, diaphoretic, hypnotic, narcotic, sedative, vasodilator and are also used in the treatment of women's complaints.

An extract of the plant depresses the motor nerves of the spinal cord, it is also slightly sedative, slightly reduces blood pressure and increases respiratory rate.

The plant contains alkaloids and flavonoids that are an effective non-addictive sedative that does not cause drowsiness. The plant is not recommended for use during pregnancy. A poultice of the roots is applied to boils, cuts, earaches, etc.

Passionflower is abundant throughout an extensive range, so it's not under threat as a species. Native tribes have used the roots as a poultice to draw out inflammation in wounds, and root teas to treat ear infections and ear aches as well as to wean infants.

(NARROW LEAF) PLANTAIN

Plantago Lanceolata

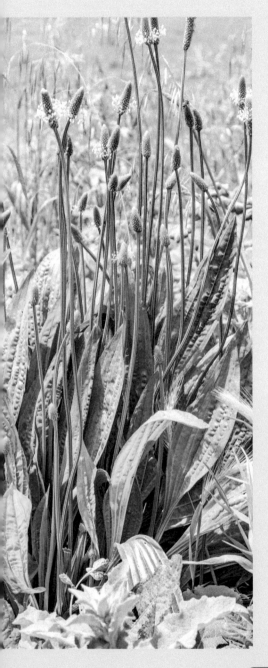

Identification

Leaves grow in a cluster, or rosette, at ground level. Leaves are broad and oval with a waxy surface and several pronounced veins parallel to the margins.

Small, white-petaled flowers are produced along the length of leafless stalks from June to September. Stalks grow 5 to 15 inches high.

Here in the South, Narrow Leaf Plantain seems to be more abundant than the Broadleaf version.

When to harvest

Plantains come back up during early spring and though the leaves can be harvested pretty early, it's best to wait until the plant goes to flower.

Fun Fact

The genus name Plantago comes from the Greek word planta, which translates to "footprint".

The broadleaf plantain is thought to look like the sole of a foot

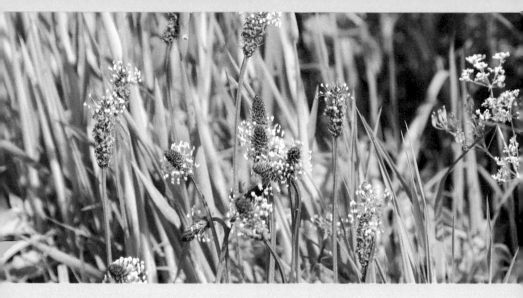

Summary

Plantain has long been considered by herbalists to be a useful remedy for coughs, wounds, inflamed skin or dermatitis, and insect bites. Bruised or crushed leaves have been applied topically to treat insect bites and stings, eczema, and small wounds or cuts. Despite being considered a weed, the common garden plantain has edible leaves and seeds.

Plantain has anti-inflammatory and astringend properties that make it useful in many medical applications, Topically, you can chew up platain leaves to make a poultice (moist mass of herbs) that can be put on minor cuts, insect bites and rashes. Internally you can make a plantain tea to fight coughs and colds.

Plantain fiber has been shown efffective in blocking intestinal pathogens from adhereing to the gut lining. It's also considered pre-biotic in nature, which means it feeds good gut bacteria, which helps promote a healthy microbiome. Plantain contains chemicals that might help decrease pain and swelling, decrease mucous, and open airways.

(LONG LEAF) PINE
Pinus Palustris

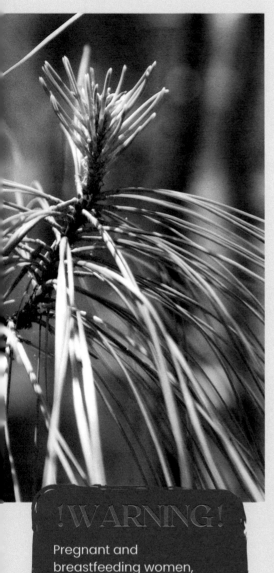

Identification

The surest way to identify conifers is to examine the needles and cones along with the bark. In general the bark of pine trees is smooth on young trees but develops a flaky, reddish-brown color with age.

Though the Southeast US is home to multiple pine species, the long leaf pine is most common.

When to harvest

Pine can be harvested any time of the year. Due to it's multiple uses it simply depends on what end product you are looking for. Fresh needles are available all year long. However, I also like to collect pine pollen in the spring, as well as pine tips. Sap is best collected in the fall to assure we're in line with nature.

Fun Fact

Several pine tree species are toxic including ponderosa pine, common yew, and Norfolk Island pine. These plants contain toxins that can cause anything from cramps to liver damage.

Those pokey needles pack large amounts of Vitamin A, as well as four-to-five times the amount of Vitamin C found in a lemon or glass of pure orange juice.

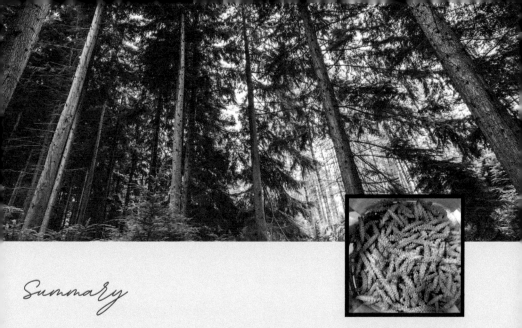

Summary

Pine needles have been used for thousands of years including in traditional chinese medicine, where pine needle tincture is used to improve digestion, reduce inflammation, and manage pain.

Hippocrates, the famous Greek father of medicine, used pine needle teas way back in 400BC for bacterial infection and to support immune function. In ancient Egypt, people would add pine needles to their cooking to kill food bacteria. In turkish folk medicine, pinus species have been used to treat rheumatic pain and for wound healing.

The simple addition of a pine needle tincture or tea into your daily routine can help aid the body in cleansing many free radicals and other bacteria that can build up and produce disease.

In modern medicine, pine needle tincture is sometimes used as an astringent to help heal wounds and skin infections. It may also be used as an expectorant to help thin mucus in the lungs. Finally, pine needle essential oil has been found to kill thirteen species of airborne bacteria.

Pine needle tea defends you against coughs and colds, improves immunity, cardiovascular functions, skin and eye health with each cup you brew. Pine needles have been used in antidepressant, antibacterial, antiviral, and inflammatory medicines.

In addition to it's many medicinal uses, pine is an excellent survival plant. The sap or resin is an excellent fire starter and makes an amazing drawing salve or bandage for first aid.

POKEWEED | POKE BERRY

Phytolacca Decandra

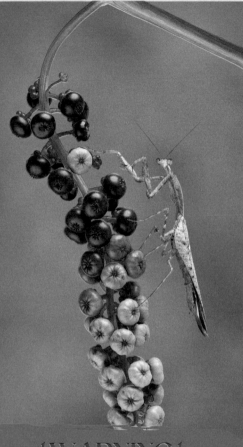

Identification

Pokeweed can grow up to 9 feet tall. Mature plants resemble shrubs or young trees. However, the stems are not woody.

When to harvest

Poke can be harvested young. The fresh shoots make good greens. Be sure they are boiled thoroughly and drained multiple times.

Berries can be harvested once completely black and dried for future use.

Fun Fact

Pokeweed is a poisonous, herbaceous plant native to the Gulf Coast of the United States. It has long been used for food and folk medicine in this part of the world and in parts of eastern North America and the Midwest.

In traditional Chinese medicine, pokeweed is known as chui xu shang lu. Due to its potential toxicity, alternative practitioners sometimes refer to it as the "Jekyll and Hyde plant."

!WARNING!

Pokeweed contains phytolaccine. This is a powerful irritant that can cause severe gastrointestinal symptoms in humans and other mammals.

Every part of the pokeweed plant is poisonous, including the roots, stems, leaves, and berries. Older plants contain higher concentrations of phytolaccine. The berries are more poisonous when green.

DO NOT USE UNLESS YOU ARE AN EXPERIENCED FORAGER AND HERBALIST

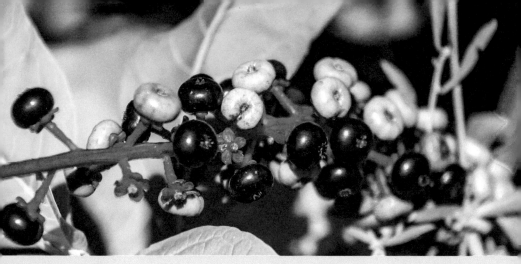

Summary

Pokeweed is also widely knows as American Nightshade, cancer root, inkberry, and pigeon berry. Many traditional cultures believe that it helps "cleanse" the body.

Historically, indigenous Americans had two main uses for pokeweed:
- As a purgative (to stimulate bowel clearance)
- As an emetic (to promote vomiting)

Poke salad is a traditional Southern dish made from the young shoots of the plant and has its origins in Native American cuisine. It's made edible by cooking the young shoots of the plant repeatedly to remove the poisonous toxins. When cooked this way, it has a flavor similar to asparagus.

Pokeweed's use in folk medicine can be traced back to a book written in the late 19th century called King's American Dispensary. This book mentioned pokeweed as a treatment for skin diseases and joint pain.

Many of pokeweed's purported benefits are attributed to a compound called pokeweed antiviral protein (PAP). Proponents believe PAP can improve skin conditions and prevent or treat viral infections.

Pokeweed berries are also used to produce dyes and are often found as an additive for coloration in wines.

PRICKLY PEAR

Opuntia Ficus-Indica

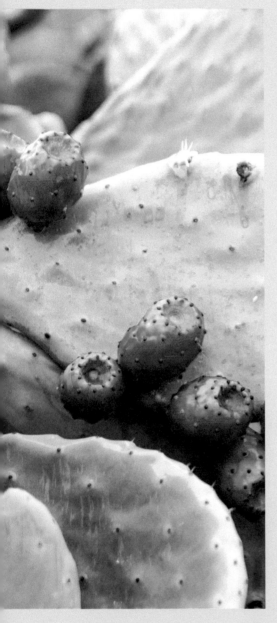

Identification

The stem of a prickly pear cactus is generally flat and broad, and it grows in segments known as pads. These pads can vary in size and shape, depending on the species. Some may have long, oval pads, while others may have rounder or more irregularly shaped ones. The pads are typically thick and fleshy and are covered in spines and small clusters of fine hairs.

When to harvest

Prickly pear is native, spreads easily, and grows year-round in our area. Therefore it can be harvested fresh at any time, either for nopales or for the fruit.

Fun Fact

The small, oval fruit that grows on top of nopales is the actual prickly pear, also known as tuna. It varies in color and can be green, pink, red, purple, or yellow-orange

This plant is a survivor! It does well in arid, and dry climates, but also in wet and steamy climates like ours, In addition it's cold hardy!

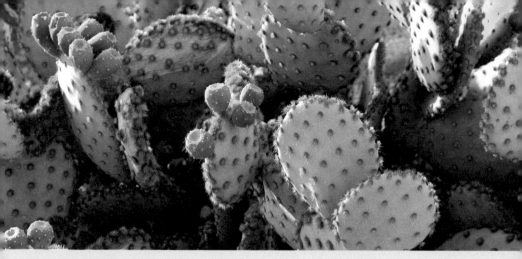

Summary

Uses of prickly pear are varied and many. Its primary use to humans is as food. The young pads are stripped of their spines, boiled and eaten as nopalitos; its use as a vegetable is widespread in Mexico and the Southwest, and has been one of the most important sources of food in this area since ancient times. The fruit is also eaten in various ways and is quite nutritious. Both are good sources of dietary fiber.

Another common use of the nopal is for natural, low-maintenance, edible fencing. Using a spine-burner, prickly pears can be made into livestock forage during droughts. The sticky sap has many uses, including use as a natural lubricant for machinery. The nopal has many traditional medicinal uses, and in modern times has been much studied for its ability to help control blood sugar levels in diabetics.

Because of its importance as food and medicine, as well as its unique appearance, the nopal has acquired much symbolic value. One appears on the flag of Mexico.

Studies suggest prickly pear may help with weight loss, promote skin and hair health, improve blood sugar and blood fat levels, and protect the liver.

As with all plant based medicinal and edible plants, prickly pear is a great addition to any diet and provides important nutritional value with it's macro nutrients, including niacin, riboflavin, vitamin B6, copper, iron, vitamin C, vitamin K, calcium, potassium, magnesium, and manganese, as well as fiber content.

RED CLOVER
Trifolium Pratense

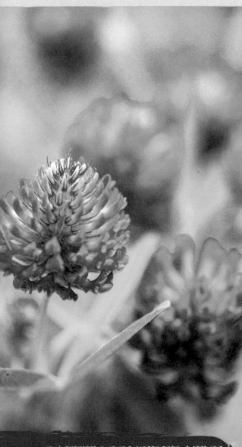

Identification

Clovers live in temperate and subtropical parts of North and South America and the Old World.

The genus name refers to the distinctive leaves, which are typically trifoliate, meaning that they have three leaflets. Some species of clover have up to nine leaflets.

There are no known poisonous look-alikes

When to harvest

Another spring flowering plant, clover can be harvested as flowers go to bloom. Just be sure to let plenty go to seed to assure bountiful harvests for years to come.

Fun Fact

There are 16 species of trifolium in Florida, but only two are native to the state.

Most of the clovers found in the Southeast United States are exotic species that have escaped from cultivation and now live in disturbed sites like pastures and roadsides.

SAFETY CONSIDERATION

Clover supplements are largely accepted to be safe for long term use.
However, they shouldn't be used by pregnant or breastfeeding women.
Clover is also not considered safe for children.
Caution should be used with individuals who are prescribed blood thinners or are actively under hormone therapy.

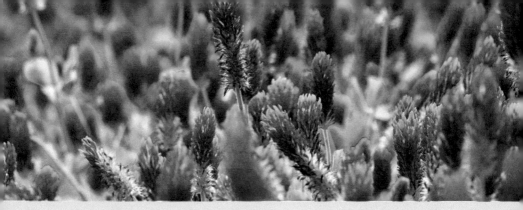

Summary

Different clover varieties are widely used in agriculture as cover or forage crop.

Within Ayurveda, trifolium pratense is believed to help remove obstructions, to be antispasmodic (can help to control some symptoms of gut spasm, muscle pain and cramps), an expectorant, a sedative, to be anti-inflammatory and an antidermatosis agent.

The flowering portion of red clover is used decoratively as an edible garnish or extract, and it can be extracted into essential oils.

Finally, it's widely used as a traditional medicine to treat osteoporosis, heart disease, arthritis, skin disorders, cancer, respiratory problems like asthma, and women's health issues, such as menstrual and menopausal symptoms. There is some evidence it may reduce the frequency of hot flashes in menopausal women.

When treating minor wounds and burns, red clover is made into an infusion or a tincture, and applied to the injured area or used as part of a poultice treatment.

Red clover is most often consumed as either a hot or cold tea or a lemonde when consumed to treat internal health issues.

The clover can be turned into a flour, and used as both a baking and cooking additive.

SPIDERWORT
Tradescantia

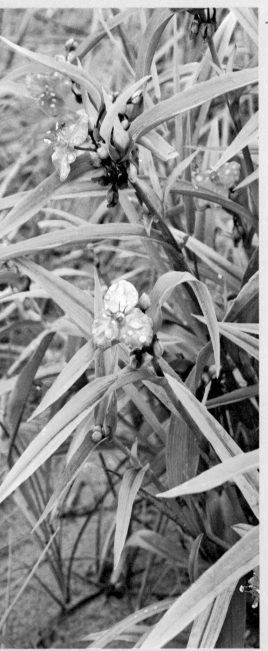

Identification

Spiderworts grow in erect clumps that can reach up to 2 feet in height. This is a perennial plant that flowers anywhere from May to October. Seeds ripen between August and October and the flowers are generally a bright blue.

Leaves tend to wrap around the stem. They are dark green and can grow to lengths of almost a foot long. Spiderwort is found growing in woodlands, hillsides, stream banks, hillsides and in moist prairies

When to harvest

This is a perennial herb and can be harvested any time of year, depending on the intended use, whether it's leaves, flowers, or seeds.

Fun Fact

Spiderwort flowers are an excellent nectar source for hummingbirds and butterflies. Butterflies love to warm their bodies up in the sun, so planting Spiderwort in sunnier areas will help maximize butterfly sightings.

Speaking of flowers: Each spiderwort flower bud blooms for a single day. But don't worry—each flower has so many buds that this singular bloom timing helps the plant appear in flower for weeks.

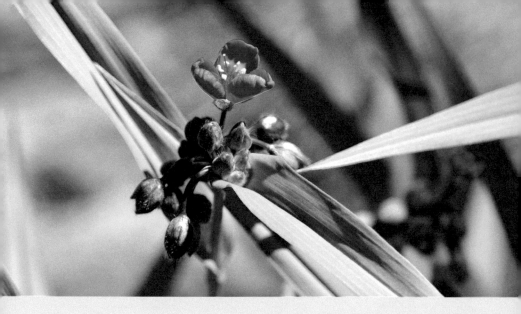

Summary

Tradescantia is a genus of 85 species of herbaceous perennial wildflowers in the family Commelinaceae, native to the Americas. Members of the genus are known by many common names, including inchplant, wandering jew, spiderwort, or dayflower.

Spiderwort had many uses in Native culture as food and medicine. The seeds are edible when roasted and ground into a powder. Leaves can be made into a tea or added to salads, soups, stews, etc. for added nutrition. tems and leaves can be steamed or sauteed like asparagus.

Roots can be collected all year round and are a laxative. They are also used as a tea in the treatment of kidney and stomach ailments and female complaints. A poultice of the leaves is applied to stings, insect bites and cancers.

Spiderwort is a Florida native edible and medicinal plant that is tolerant of the intense summer heat. The entire plant is edible and has many different uses. You will find spiderwort blossoming year round in Florida, but the height of its bloom is in the spring. Energetically, spiderwort is a cooling, soothing plant.

The fresh leaves and stems can be made into a poultice and used topically to relieve inflamed skin conditions, similar to Aloe vera.

STINGING NETTLE
Urtica Dioica

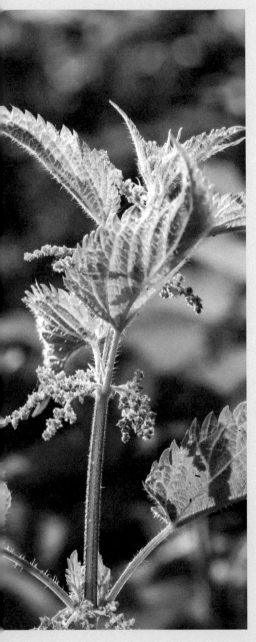

Identification

Nettles grow 2 to 5 feet tall and have opposite leaves. The leaves are coarsely toothed, pointed on the ends, and can be several inches long.

They are considered invasive, as they stem from Europe and will agressively take over native areas.

Both stinging and wood nettles grow abundantly in our area, are in the mint family and distinguish themselves via their stinging hairs from other mints.

When to harvest

Spring is big for harvesting wild plants. You can find new growth nettles early to late spring pretty much everywhere you look. Be sure to wear gloves when harvesting.

Fun Fact

A mature nettle is amazingly fibrous. The fiber content of nettles makes this plant an outstanding source to produce clothing. In fact one hectare of plants will yield enough fiber to make 100 shirts.

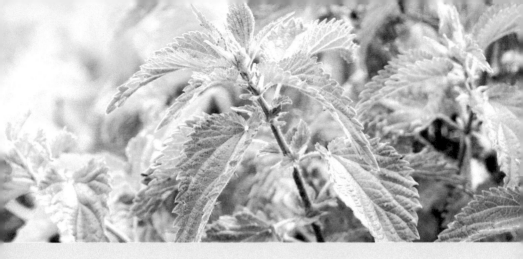

Summary

Stinging nettle has antiproliferative, anti-inflammatory, antioxidant, analgesic, anti-infectious, hypotensive, and anti-ulcer characteristics, as well as the ability to prevent cardiovascular disease, in all parts of the plant: leaves, stems, roots and seeds.

Stinging nettle offers a variety of vitamins, minerals, fatty acids, amino acids, polyphenols and pigments, many of which also act as antioxidant inside your body.

In medieval Europe, it was used as a diuretic and to treat joint pain. Stinging nettle has fine hairs on the leaves and stems that contain irritating chemicals, which are released when the plant comes in contact with the skin.

For centuries, nettle has been a staple for ancient cultures and continues to be an important food source throughout the world.

It's arguably one of the most nutritional wild edibles available, but it needs to be cooked or dried to neutralize the sting.

Stinging nettle grows in such abundance, that over-harvesting is not really an issue. With it's multitude of applications and nutritional value it should be a staple in any diet.

SWEET GUM
Liquidambar Styraciflua

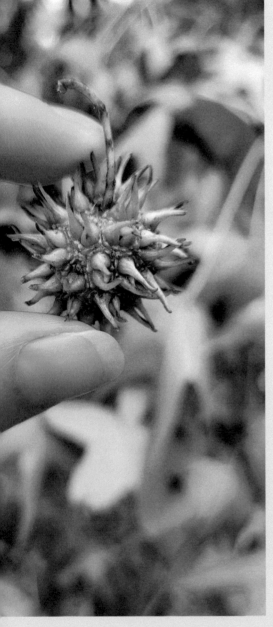

Identification

Sweet gum grows into a large tree. Leaves are alternate, simple, star-shaped, with 5 lobes. A tell-tale sign on whether you have sweet gum on your property will be the spikey seed pods, which are plenty.

Although sweetgum trees have attracted widespread use in landscaping, most sweetgum trees are found growing as a volunteer species among commercial pine forests that are cultivated for the softwood lumber and pulpwood industries.

When to harvest

Finally, a plant for fall! Sweet Gum trees produce seed pods, which should be harvested when green during early fall. The medicinal properties lay with the infertile seeds. Once matured, the seed pods make for great dried decorations!

Fun Fact

Settlers and soldiers could peel back the bark to expose the liquorish flavored sap so they could chew it like gum. This is why it has the name sweetgum.

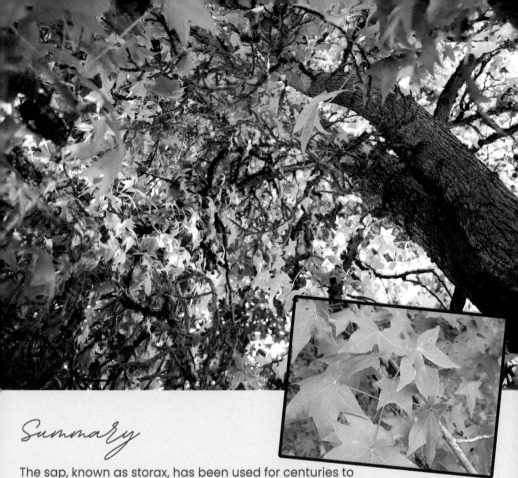

Summary

The sap, known as storax, has been used for centuries to treat common ailments such as skin problems, coughs, and ulcers. More recently, storax has proven to be a strong antimicrobial agent even against multi-drug resistant bacteria.

The infertile seeds found in each of the sweet gum's compound seed capsules are a naturally occurring source of shikimic acid, one of the main ingredients in the manufacture of flu medication.

Storax has medicinal uses dating back to the Aztec Empire. The ancient Aztecs collected the boiled down sap, and used it as a treatment for skin infections and other ailments.

Native tribes and nations also used storax for medicinal purposes, including controlling coughs and dysentery and treating sores and wounds. In addition to storax, the sap of the sweetgum tree was burnt as incense or mixed with tobacco leaves as a sedative as well as used in the making of soaps, cosmetics, fixatives in perfumes, adhesives, and lacquers

TURKEY TAIL

Trametes Versicolor

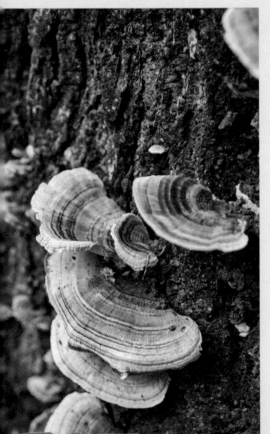

Identification

Turkey Tail mushrooms typically grow on dead trees, but have a few look-alikes which do not carry the same medicinal properties.

To properly identify turkey tail, check the clear coloring as well as the underside of the mushroom, which should have tiny pores, no gills.

When to harvest

Once fungi reach maturity, they go past prime harvesting time very quickly. Turkey tail is best harvested fresh.

Fun Fact

As long as you don't mind your mushrooms leathery and hardly chewable, they are edible.

While turkey tail mushrooms are not toxic, they are not exactly a culinary delight. However, they make a great addition to dishes, shakes or even coffee in powdered form.

SAFETY CONSIDERATION

Because turkey tail is a fungus, anyone with a mushroom or mold allergy should not use it.

Taking any mushroom extract could cause a life threatening reaction in some people.

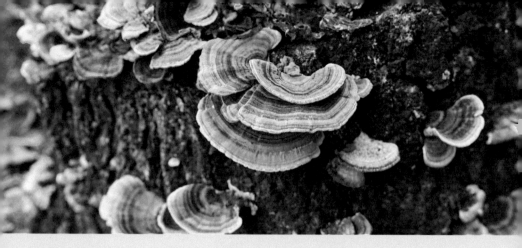

Summary

Turkey tail is a medicinal mushroom with an impressive range of benefits. It contains a variety of powerful antioxidants and other compounds that may help boost your immune system and even help fight certain cancers. Plus, turkey tail may improve gut bacteria balance, which can positively impact your immunity.

A few of the traditional uses for turkey tail include: removing toxins, increasing energy, removing excessive fluid, strengthening the organs responsible for the immune system, and supporting liver, lung and spleen function. Some conditions that benefit from turkey tail use include coughs, breathing difficulties, hemorrhoids and joint pain.

Turkey tail mushrooms are rich in antioxidant compounds, helping the body fight free radicals and adapt to oxidative stress.

In conventional medicine, turkey tail has been used to support the immune systems of people.

Turkey tail has prebiotic abilities and helps the gut regulate its balance of bacteria. Prebiotics are a type of fiber that act as a food source for healthy bacteria in the gut.

USNEA (OLD MAN'S BEARD)

Usnea Filipendula

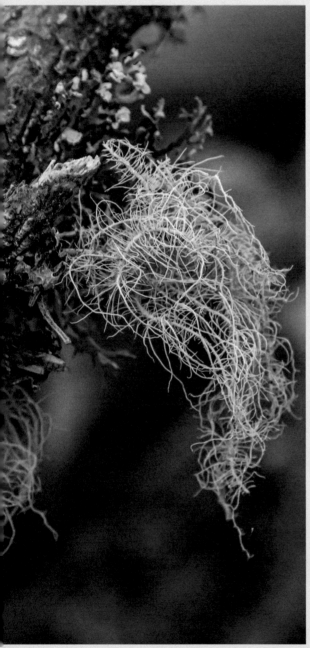

Identification

As a lichen, usnea grows on trees and is often found on oaks. Usnea has an elastic center and is easily identified by giving it a slight pull, where it will reveal an elastic white or silver center.

When to harvest

Usnea can be harvested any time of year. However, avoid picking usnea off trees directly as it is very slow growing. Best harvesting practice for usnea dictates to pick it off the ground after a hard rain storm.

Fun Fact

Though it looks similar to Spanish Moss to the untrained eye, they are very different.

Where usnea is a lichen, Spanish Moss is actually an air plant, in the same plant family as pineapple!

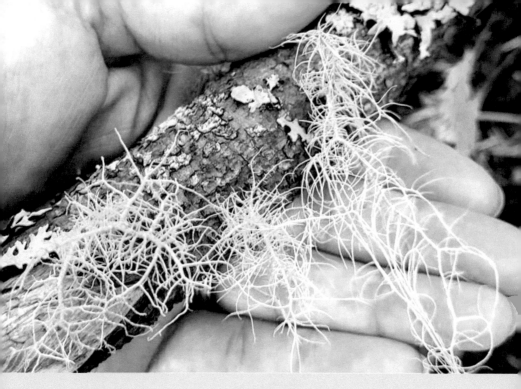

Summary

Although usnea is also considered a tonic, this lichen is an infection fighter, plain and simple. Unlike most modern antibiotics which disrupt the structure of a cell, this lichen prevents the metabolism of bacteria.

It has been successfully used to treat certain type of infections, such as those affecting the throat, respiratory tract, mouth, urinary tract, and skin wounds that wont easily heal. It is particularly effective for hot, irritable, wet coughs, and can support weight loss, due to its potential ability to support metabolic processes.

As an herbal support it is often used by itself or as an added fighter within other herbal applications.

Usnea contains a chemical called usnic acid (sodium usniate) that might cause liver damage if used extensively over long time periods.

Because usnea is very slow growing, it should only be harvested off fallen limbs to ensure sustainable and ethical foraging.

(WILD) VIOLET
Viola Sororia Priceana

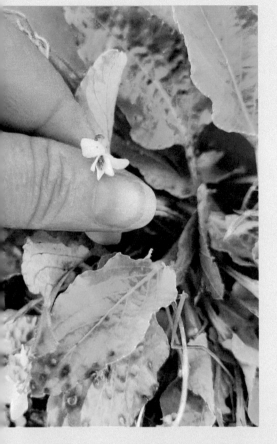

Identification

Leaves are basal, heart-shaped, many solitary, 1 inch flowers on slender stalks.

Herbaceous plant with purple to white spring flowers. Violets grow as a perennial in our area and spread similarly to mints both via seeds and rhizomes.

When to harvest

Violets are everywhere during early spring and will die back once temperatures in the South get a bit too warm for them. You can harvest violets for both flowers and leaves once they are in bloom.

Fun Fact

Viola odorata is used as a source for scents in the perfume industry. Violet is known to have a 'flirty' scent as its fragrance comes and goes.
A chemical present in the flowers turns off the ability for humans to smell the fragrant compound for moments at a time.

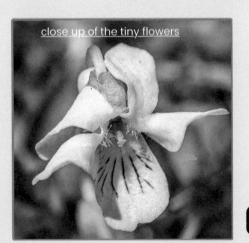

close up of the tiny flowers

75

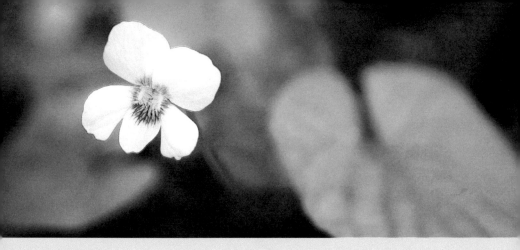

Summary

The leaves and flowers of the common blue violet, along with many other species, are edible and medicinal. The "confederate violet" is commonly found as a wild and escaped cultivar. It has white flowers with blue streaks and is an inhabitant of lawns in the southeastern United States. Much of the American use of violets stems from the European herbal tradition.

The flowers are lettuce-like and have a subtle peppery flavor. Wild violets are a gentle herb, so it can be eaten in large quantities and is safe for people taking medicines.

Wild violets have helped treat many conditions over several centuries. The upper parts of the plant can be used as an infusion to promote sleep. Taken in a strong tea, they help with lung health by working as an expectorant. Wild violets help treat infections in the upper respiratory tract, as well as colds, congestion, flu viruses, and bronchitis. Overall, they are a gentle immune system stimulant.

Violet is cooling and moistening and is used internally as a blood cleanser, respiratory remedy, and lymphatic stimulant. Violet has a rich tradition in Europe, where it has been used for centuries as a pulmonary remedy for dry, hacking cough. It is often recommended for bronchitis and whooping cough. Violet can also be used as a tonic for chronically swollen lymph nodes.

Topically, violet is used as a poultice, compress, infused oil, and salve for dry or chafed skin, abrasions, insect bites, eczema, varicose veins and more. It is cooling, soothing, and anti-inflammatory.

WILD LETTUCE

Lactuca Virosa & Lactuca Serriola

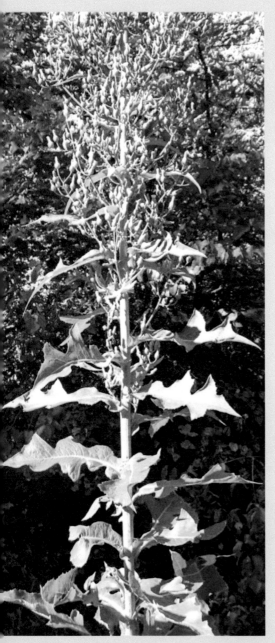

Identification

Wild lettuce is a weedy biennial plant. Usually growing as a basal rosette in its first year, then sending up a stalk and flowering in its second year.

Exudes white milky latex. Has hair of the underside of each leaf along the midrib. Midrib cross-section shape is triangular.

Flowers come in various colors, though in our area they tend to most commonly be yellow.

When to harvest

Wild lettuce should be harvested during the second year, when it will grow up to 9 foot tall. I recommend harvesting after it has set flowers.

Fun Fact

Wild lettuce is a powerful herbal pain reliever, hence why the plant is often called "opium lettuce."

While the plant will relieve pain, don't expect the hardcore sedative effects of opium. It is more comparable to a high dosage of ibuprofen.

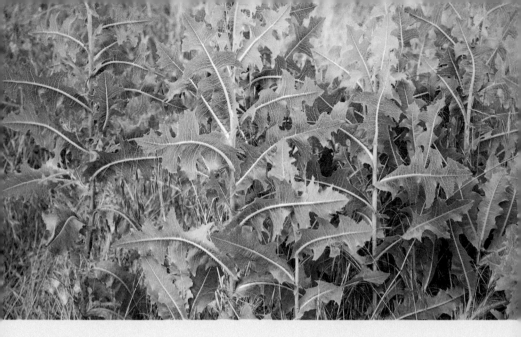

Summary

Both Lactuca Virosa and Lactuca Serriola can be used interchangeably for pain relief. It is generally accepted that the virosa is more potent, although I can find no scientific source to back this up.

Wild lettuce has several prominent historical medicinal uses in addition to being a choice of edible greens! Many people seek this plant out in order to use it for medicinal purposes today.

It's been studied for sedative and pain-relieving effects and for managing stress and chronic pain, and is also used as a sleep aid.

The components which provide pain relief are known as lactones. They act on the central nervous system to calm the nerves which cause pain sensations.

All plant parts contain the active medicinal components. However, these components are low in young plants. Thus, it is best to harvest from adult plants in the second year of growth, right after its flowering period.

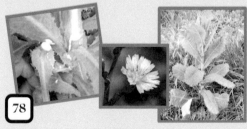

(COASTALPLAIN) WILLOW

Salix Caroliniana

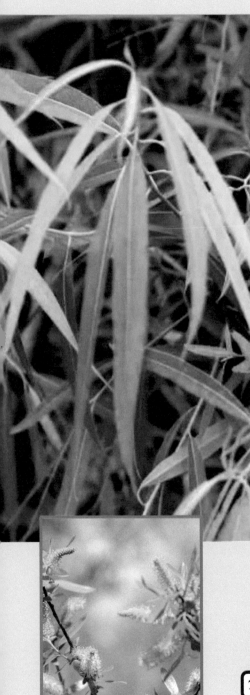

Identification

This tree can be attractive most of the year due to its fairly fine leaves. It is at its best for a brief period in early spring when it blooms and then sets masses of white fruit at a time when little else is blooming.

When to harvest

Though you could technically harvest leaves and boil them down into a green mass, it would take massive seasoning and preparation to make them somewhat edible.

However, what we are really after with willows, is the bark of the tree, which can be harvested any time of the year. For the medicinal compound we want to harvest the inner bark, to be specific.

Fun Fact

It is a moisture-loving plant and is found along the edges of bodies of water, in marshes and wet forests. It can be shrubby or it can grow to tree stature. The largest coastalplain willow on record is 52 feet tall, with a crown spread of nearly 53 feet in Alachua County, Florida.

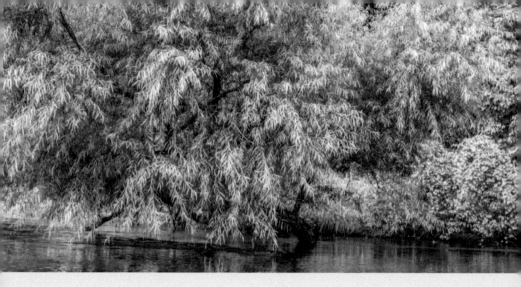

Summary

The Coastalplain Willow is the only willow tree native to our area, and it thrives in moist and wet environments, which make it a perfect fit for the swamps of Florida.

Mention willow, and aspirin comes to mind. Literally for thousands of years, humans have turned to the bark of this tree to treat a variety of ailments — headaches, fever and the like. In fact coastalplain willow, Salix caroliana, is known as the toothache tree because of its analgesic qualities. All of this is because of salicin compounds that willows possess.

If you decide to try it out and chew some of the bark, be careful, as it will numb your mouth.

Both the Houma tribe of Louisiana and the Seminoles used coastalplain willow extensively for a variety of medicinal purposes — breaking fevers, alleviating aches and pains, headaches and other complaints.

The first clinical study on willow bark was done in 1763 and showed that it could be used to treat malaria. Since then, there have been hundreds of clinical studies testing the benefits of willow bark, including treatment for fever, pain, arthritis, headaches and other inflammatory conditions. Willow bark has also recently become very popular for treating acne and is found in many skin products.

WOOD SORREL

Oxalis

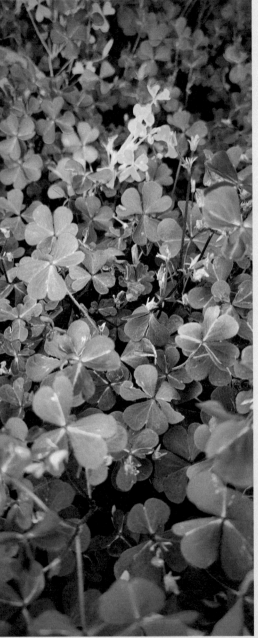

Identification

Wood sorrel is a genus of flowering plants composed of over 500 species that grow around the globe. In North America we have numerous species, including Oxalis stricta. On my land I also have the violacea version, which adds a nice splash of color.

When to harvest

Sorrels are extremely prolific and in our area will grow everywhere all year long. It makes for a great groundcover, when you need quick coverage as well. Due to its prolific nature, this little plant can be harvested whenever you would like it freshly. There should be no need to harvest and preserve through dehydration or other methods.

Fun Fact

The sour flavor is a result of oxalic acid, which can cause problems with nutrient absorption if taken in very large quantities, but it's unlikely you'd eat enough wood sorrel to experience difficulty.

Oxalic acid is found in many common foods, including chocolate, coffee, beets, and dark leafy greens like spinach.

People with arthritis, gout, or a history of kidney stones are advised to limit their consumption of oxalic acid.

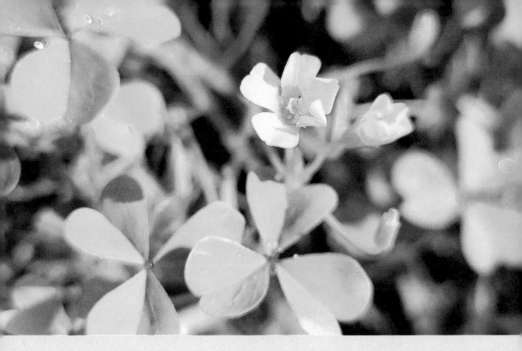

Summary

Wood Sorrel, also know as sour grass, which is very fitting, has a tart, lemony taste, and the whole plant is edible. As with most edible plants, it also has medicinal properties and benefits. The plant can be steeped in hot water to make tea. Because Yellow Wood Sorrel is high in vitamin C, it has been used to treat scurvy, liver, and digestive disorders.

Wood sorrels are a terrific choice for beginner foragers, easy to identify and beloved by kiddos for its lemony flavor. Its signature heart-shaped leaves have led to one of its other nicknames, lemon hearts. You may also have heard it called sourgrass, common yellow oxalis, sheep's clover, lemon clover, shamrock, or other regional variations.

It tends to pop up everywhere, including in the garden beds, where I just leave it alone and pull it alongside whatever we are harvesting that day.

It has diuretic and refrigerant action, and a decoction made from it can be a great solution for feverish kids, both for hydration as well as to lower the fever. It's also a favorite to brew for intestinal complaints as it strengthens the stomache, entices appetite, curbs vomiting and helps with abdominal pain and constipation. As a gargle it helps remedy mouth ulcers. It also assists with wound healing, staunch bleeding, and reduces swelling and inflammation.

YAUPON HOLLY
Ilex Vomitoria

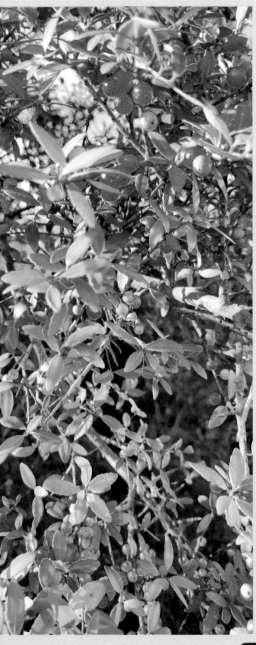

Identification

Yaupon is a native, perennial, evergreen shrub capable of reaching approximately 30 feet in height under ideal conditions.
The bark is smooth, light grey with lighter grey to nearly white splotches. The leaves are alternate and oval in shape. They are dark green with a leathery appearance and a lighter colored underside.
It's a species of holley and produces the tell-tale bright red berries during fall and winter.

When to harvest

Yaupon is an evergreen shrub and the leaves can therefore be harvested all year long. Young growth during the spring growth spurt will make for a more subtle aroma, whereas older growth will add some bitterness to the leaves.
The berries are not recommended for harvesting as they can cause very heavy digestive discomfort and potential hospitalization.

Fun Fact

Yaupon got its unfortunate Latin name from European colonists, who gave yaupon the ill-sounding scientific name Ilex vomitoria due to its use in purging rituals.

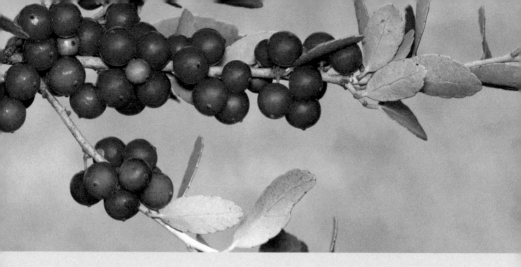

Summary

Yaupon tea is an herbal tea known for its medicinal properties. It boasts a unique flavor and rich nutrient profile, packing plenty of antioxidants and beneficial compounds into each serving. Plus, it may also offer several benefits and help promote brain function, decrease inflammation, and support healthy energy levels.

Yaupon tea is a natural source of caffeine, which can comprise up to 2% of the tea's dry weight. With that in mind yaupon has around 1/3 less caffeine then coffee.

It also contains theobromine, a compound that may improve focus and brain function, and is rich in several polyphenols, which are natural compounds that act as antioxidants to reduce inflammation and prevent oxidative damage to your cells.

You may come across many other names for the yaupon plant, such as Cassine, Appalachian tea, South-Sea tea, or Christmas-berry tree. The leaves can be used fresh, dried or roasted, which results in different tasting brews.

Today, besides being used as a nourishing herbal tea, yaupon also serves as a common ingredient in skincare products like cleaners, moisturizers, and serums.

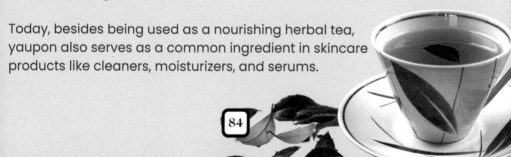

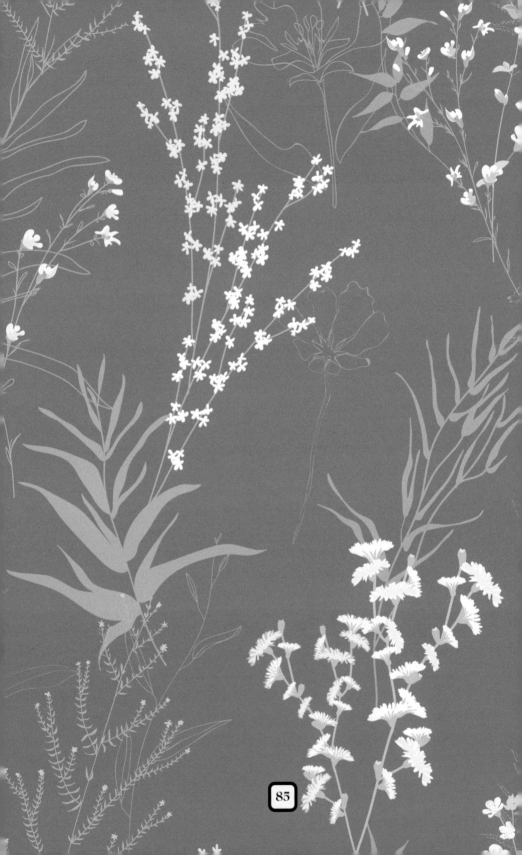

CHAPTER 4

Favorite Recipes and Preparations

GENERAL OVERVIEW

Though teas are probably the simplest herbal preparation method, I also like tincturing and infusing oils for lotions and salves.

Teas can be hot or cold brewed, depending on if you need a cup immediately or for later use. In general, when brewing a hot cup, 4-6 minutes of infusion is typically enough. However, for cold brewing tea you will need to use a bit more botanical material as well as letting it infuse for a minimum 6 hours. I usually shoot for 12.

As a rule of thumb when infusing oils or tincturing botanical material, use a 1:1 ratio for fresh herbs. For dried herbs, use a 1-4 ratio.

To infuse oils use a high quality carrier oil. "Virgin" oils are best as they are cold-pressed and therefore retain the highest amount of their natural benefits. Oils derived via heat processing can loose much of their initial benefits.

Olive, Argan, Jojoba, Coconut, Sweet Almond, Rosehip Seed, Hemp Seed, Avocado, Safflower, and Grapeseed Oil are generally accepted to be the best. However, if you are dealing with tree nut allergies, you should forego oils derived from them.

The most common medium for tincturing is alcohol. That's because it's an effective preservative and powerful extractor. I recommend using a clear 80proof alcohol, such as vodka or Everclear. Dark alcohols can have traces of other ingredients you may not want in your tinctures.

If you would like to stay away from alcohol; glycerin, vinegar, and vegetable glycerol are the preferred solvents for alcohol-free tinctures. Glycerin is sweet, making it ideal for herbs with a bitter taste, while vinegar provides a tangy flavor. Vegetable glycerol is a popular choice due to its neutral taste. Choose the solvent that best complements the herbs you have selected.

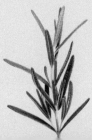
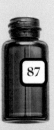
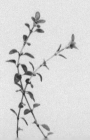
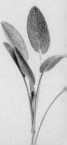

INFUSED OILS

1. Place dried herbs in a dry, sterilized container and cover with the appropriate amount of room-temperature oil.
2. Use a dry, sterilized spoon to mix thoroughly so all surfaces of the herb(s) are coated with oil and no air bubbles remain.
3. Place a square piece of natural waxed paper on top of the jar, then seal jar with a lid (this protects the herbal oil from any chemical coating that may be on the lid)

There are a number of ways you can infuse your oils. Though I personally use the folk and solar methods, I am including other ways you can make your own as well.

To create an herb-infused oil using the **folk method,** simply fill a dry, sterilized container with dried herbs and pour room-temperature oil over the herbs, making sure to completely cover the herbs. Let infuse for 4-6 weeks in a warm, dark place,

For "solar" infusion: Once your herbs and oils have been combined in the jar and sealed, place the jar in a brown paper bag or wrap it in an opaque cloth, and place it in a sunny window sill or directly in the sunlight for 1-2 weeks.

For both the folk and solar method, shake the jar every few days to assure herbs and oil are combining nicely. This helps with extracting all the goodness into your carrier oil.

For "double-boiler infusion": Begin by placing a stainless steel saucepan on the stove, filling it ¼ full of water, and bringing the water to a boil. Place your herbs and oils into a second dry, sterilized stainless steel saucepan that is slightly smaller than the first. Use a dry, sterilized spoon to mix thoroughly so all surfaces of the herb(s) are coated and no air bubbles remain. Place the smaller, herb-filled saucepan inside the larger, water-filled saucepan and simmer for 30-60 minutes, keeping a careful eye on the amount of water in the larger pan and being very careful not to let water splash into the oil/herb mixture. Monitor the temperature of your oil and keep it between 120-140 degrees Fahrenheit. If the water level runs low in the lower saucepan, carefully add more hot water to bring the water level in the saucepan back up to ¼ full.

The double boiler method is the quickest way to get your finished product and you can strain immediately.

TINCTURES

To prepare the extraction medium, mix one part herb (by weight) with four parts of your chosen solvent. If you prefer a stronger tincture, increase the herb-to-solvent ratio. Place the mixture in a glass jar and ensure that all the plant material is submerged. Seal the jar tightly and shake it gently to promote proper mixing.

After preparing the extraction medium, the next step is the extraction process itself.

Label and date your jar: It's important to keep track of your tincture's creation date and ingredients used.

Infusion period: Place your jar in a cool, dark place for 2-4 weeks for vinegar or alcohol-based tinctures, or 4-6 weeks for glycerin-based tinctures. Shake gently every few days.

Straining: After the infusion period, strain the liquid through a fine mesh strainer or cheesecloth, pressing the herbs to extract all the liquid. I usually feed the leftover plant material to our chickens or pigs.

Storage: Transfer the strained liquid into amber glass dropper bottles for storage. Remember to label each bottle with the herb and creation date.

Shelf life: Alcohol-free tinctures generally have a shorter shelf life than alcohol-based ones. Store your glycerin tinctures in a cool, dark place. They don't need to be refrigerated and can last 3-5 years. Vinegar tinctures are best stored in the refrigerator, where they will keep for up to a year.

SALVES

Salves are an herbal preparation made from herb infused carrier oil and bees wax. This, of course, is the most basic salve and many variations are possible.

A ratio of 4:1 to 8:1 is generally recommended, which translates to 1 part of beeswax to 4 parts of infused oil, and so on.

I have found that with our Southern heat and humidity, the best ratio tends to be in the 4:1 to 5:1 range, as it provides a higher melting point.

Should you prefer the consistency of a lotion or body butter over a salve for general skin care, I recommend adding shea butter to the mix, or adding water and "whipping" up a batch of body lotion or butter.

Shelf life for a salve is generally 12+ months, whereas a lotion should ideally be refrigerated and used within 2-3 months.

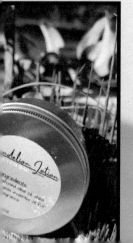
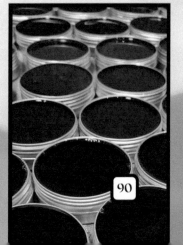
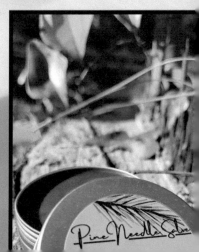

TEAS & SIMPLE INFUSIONS

Teas are the simplest preparation for herbal material.

A great benefit of loose leaf tea is the fact that you can mix and match to your preferred taste and can adjust to any needs you may have.

When brewing tea, whether it is by the cup or by the gallon, I suggest sweetening with local honey after the brew is complete for additional health benefits.

When mixing and matching your preferred brews, I recommend having some basic herbals such as chamomile and peppermint on hand as they make a great base for any tea if this is a new adventure for you. In addition, it is smart to keep fresh or dried lemons or oranges at hand for an extra kick of Vitamin C and taste.

The tea recipes following are listed with my preferred blending ratios. However, you can easily adjust these to fit your own needs.

IMMUNE SUPPORT TEA

1 cup Elderberry
1 cup Blackberry Leaf
1/4 cup Brown Eyed Susan
1/4 cup Pine Needle
2 Tbsp Usnea

GOOD-NIGHT TEA

1 cup Chamomile
1/2 cup Blackberry Leaf
1/2 cup Wild Violet

DIGESTIVE TEA

1 cup Peppermint
1/4 cup Dandelion Root
1/4 cup Plantain
1/4 cup Wood Sorrel

LIFT YOUR SPIRITS TEA

1 cup Lemon Balm
1/2 cup Blackberry Leaf
2 Tbsp Mimosa

WOMEN'S HEALTH TEA

1 cup Blackberry Leaf
1 cup Elderflower
1/4 cup Red Clover

FIRE CIDER

Fire cider is a potent herbal tonic and has been a staple in holistic health for decades. It's packed with a variety of health-boosting ingredients, using raw apple cider vinegar as a base.

The basic recipe can be adjusted to your personal preference and it's a really fun infusion to play around with every time you make a new batch. Fire Cider is great to have on hand for cold & flu season, but is commonly recommended for continued use, due to it's general support of health and wellness. The basic ingredients bring a number of benefits to the table including:

- Immune System Support
- Anti-Inflammatory Effects
- Digestive Aid
- Circulatory Health
- Natural Decongestant
- Antioxidant Properties

Common components include garlic, ginger, horseradish, hot peppers, onions, and citrus. These ingredients are steeped together for several weeks, producing a potent elixir.

Fire cider can be taken in various ways, depending on your preference and tolerance level.

- **Straight Shot:** Take a tablespoon of fire cider straight, especially at the onset of a cold or to give your immune system a quick boost.
- **Diluted in Water:** Mix a tablespoon of fire cider in a glass of water for a more diluted, less intense flavor. You can also add some honey for taste
- **Salad Dressing:** Use fire cider as a zesty base for homemade salad dressings.
- **Marinades and Sauces:** Incorporate fire cider into marinades for meat and vegetables or add a splash to sauces for an extra kick.

NICOLE'S SIGNATURE FIRE CIDER

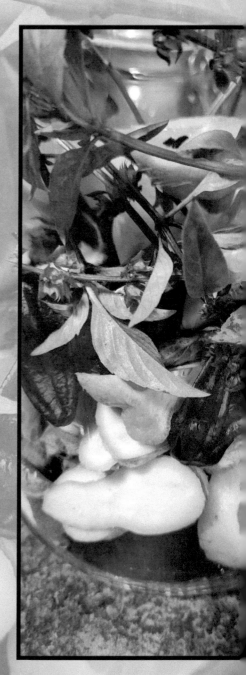

Ingredients:

4 bulbs of garlic
4 large jalapenos or chili peppers
1 large ginger root
2 fresh lemons
5-6 sprigs of Tulsi
1 cup of Hibiscus petals

Instructions:

1. Add fresh or dried prepared botanical ingredients to a half gallon mason jar.
2. Cover with raw apple cider vinegar and steep or "ferment" for 2-6 weeks.
3. Strain and bottle, preferrably in an amber bottle if on hand
4. Store strained Fire Cider in the refrigerator

Fire cider has a shelf life of 6-12 months

HERBAL POWDERS & SEASONINGS

An easy way to add herbal nutrition to your diet is through powders and seasonings.

I love creating easy to use ingredients, which will add some zing to any meal.

If you have access to a dehydrator, the steps to creating your own line of seasonings is very simple. However you do not need a dehydrator and can simply hang botanicals to dry slowly. A dehydrator just helps moving things along quicker.

1. Harvest your botanicals
2. Dehydrate (recommend 105-115F at 12-18 hours)
3. Pulverize them. I like to use an electric coffee mill.
4. Combine to your liking.

Through this method, I always have extra dehydrated nutrition on hand to add to soups, stews, shakes, and more.

PRESERVES & SYRUPS

Simple preserves and syrups are another great way to use an abundance of wild food.

Berries, such as blackberries, elderberries and beautyberries make excellent jams, jellies and syrups. Elder flowers and magnolia flowers make an excellent syrup as well as fritters.

ELDER OR MAGNOLIA FLOWER FRITTERS

1. Harvest fresh, shake out to clean (do not wash as it will cause the plant material to soften and brown)
2. Coat in egg wash and preferred coating
3. Pan fry and enjoy!

These are delicious with a side of fresh berry jam.

SIMPLE BLACKBERRY JAM

Ingredients:

4 cups fresh blackberries
2 cups granulated sugar
1 tablespoon lemon juice

Instructions:

1. Rinse the blackberries thoroughly under cool running water.
2. Drain well and mash them slightly with a potato masher or fork to release their juices.
3. In a large saucepan, combine the mashed blackberries, sugar, and lemon juice. Stir well to ensure the sugar is evenly distributed.
4. Place the saucepan over medium-high heat. Bring the mixture to a boil, stirring frequently to prevent sticking. Once boiling, reduce the heat to medium and continue to cook. Stir regularly and gently mash the berries to your desired consistency.
5. Cook the jam until it reaches the desired thickness, about 15-20 minutes. To check if the jam is ready, place a small amount on a chilled plate. If it wrinkles when you push it with your finger, it's done. If not, continue cooking for a few more minutes and test again.
6. Once the jam has reached the desired consistency, remove the saucepan from heat.
7. Carefully ladle the hot jam into sterilized jars, leaving about 1/4-inch headspace at the top. Wipe the rims of the jars with a clean, damp cloth and seal with lids.
8. Let the jars cool to room temperature. Store the jam in the refrigerator for immediate use or process in a water bath canner for longer shelf life.

ELDERFLOWER SYRUP

Ingredients:
20-25 elderflower heads
4 cups granulated sugar
2 cups water
2 lemons (preferably organic)
2 tablespoons citric acid (optional, for preservation)

Instructions:
1. Gently shake the elderflower heads to remove any insects or debris. Do not wash the flowers, as this can wash away some of the flavor. Trim the thick stems, leaving just the flowers and small stems.
2. Thinly slice the lemons. Remove any seeds to avoid bitterness.
3. Make the Syrup: In a large saucepan, combine the sugar and water. Heat gently, stirring occasionally, until the sugar has completely dissolved. Bring the syrup to a gentle boil, then remove from heat.
4. Combine Ingredients: Add the elderflower heads and lemon slices to the syrup.
5. Stir in the citric acid. Ensure all the flowers are submerged in the syrup.
6. Cover the saucepan with a clean kitchen towel or lid. Let the mixture steep for 24-48 hours at room temperature, stirring occasionally.
7. After steeping, strain the mixture through a fine-mesh sieve or cheesecloth into a large bowl or jug. Press down on the flowers and lemons to extract as much liquid as possible.
8. Pour the strained syrup into sterilized bottles or jars. Seal tightly with lids.
9. Store the elderflower syrup in the refrigerator, where it will keep for several weeks.
10. For longer storage, consider processing the bottles in a water bath canner.

Serving Suggestions:
- Mix the syrup with still or sparkling water for a refreshing drink.
- Add to cocktails for a floral twist.
- Drizzle over pancakes, waffles, or desserts.

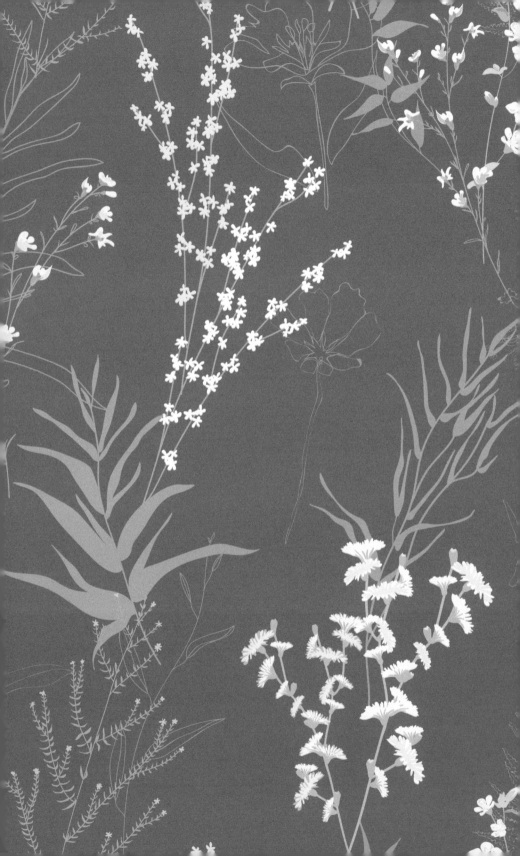

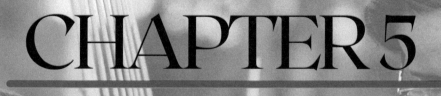

CHAPTER 5

Bonus Material

FORAGING & HOLISTIC HEALTH

Remember, using herbs to supplement your diet is a holistic approach. Incorporating botanicals into your routine helps your body heal itself naturally.

Our bodies possess an incredible ability to combat intruders with a strong immune system. Supporting it by strengthening your immune system through quality food, exercise, fresh air, and herbal supplements can improve your overall well-being and address the root causes of ailments rather than just treating symptoms.

When adding dietary supplements to your daily routine, keep in mind that there are no "spot" treatments. These supplements are designed to support overall health and well-being, helping your body respond to various bacteria, viruses, and inflammation.

FORAGING
OR CULTIVATING?

Foraged herbals and garden-grown herbs represent two distinct approaches to acquiring medicinal and culinary plants, each with its own set of advantages and considerations.

Foraged herbals involve harvesting plants from their natural habitats, such as forests, meadows, or wild landscapes. This method relies on the abundance of indigenous or wild plants that have adapted to their specific environments. In these environments, we seek out plants with medicinal properties, harnessing the knowledge of traditional herbalism.

Foraging encourages the exploration and appreciation of diverse plant species present in natural ecosystems. With wildcrafting we take a more sustainable and environmentally conscious approach, as we want to prioritize responsible harvesting to ensure the longevity of plant populations. Foraging also allows us to be connected to Mother Nature and gain firsthand knowledge about plant identification, seasons, and habitats.

Though I am a big proponent of foraging wild plants responsibly, wildcrafting comes with giving up a controlled environment and potential easy access, as we are subject to the availability and accessibility of wild plants, which can vary based on location, climate, and environmental factors.

Garden grown herbs involve cultivating plants in controlled environments, such as home gardens, community plots, or commercial farms. This method provides individuals with the ability to cultivate specific herbs for desired qualities and uses.

In our garden we have greater control over soil quality, water, and sunlight, enabling optimal growth conditions for herbs. This will usually result in a more predictable harvest, where we can plan and manage harvests, ensuring a consistent supply of herbs throughout the growing season. We can then also choose specific herb varieties, allowing for the cultivation of medicinal, culinary, or ornamental herbs tailored to individual preferences.

However, cultivated gardens may lack the diversity found in natural ecosystems, potentially limiting exposure to a broader range of plant species. Garden-grown herbs require resources like water, fertilizers, and space, which might not be as sustainable as foraging in certain contexts.

Both methods offer unique benefits and challenges, contributing to the diversity of approaches in herbalism and plant-based practices.

FORAGING
WITH THE SEASONS

In a fast-paced world dominated by supermarkets and convenience stores, reconnecting with nature's abundance through foraging can be a rewarding and sustainable way to source food. Learning about your local flora, while keeping seasons and wildlife in mind, adds a layer of responsibility and harmony to this ancient practice.

Foraging is more than just gathering wild plants; it's a profound connection with the environment. To embark on this journey, start by understanding the seasonal cycles in your region. Different plants thrive during various times of the year, and being attuned to these patterns ensures a respectful and sustainable harvest.

Spring: Look for tender young shoots, wild greens, and blossoms. Dandelions, wild garlic, and violets are often early spring delights.

Summer: This season offers a bounty of fruits, berries, and a variety of herbs. Blueberries, blackberries, and elderflowers are common finds. Be mindful of plant populations and avoid overharvesting to allow for future growth.

Fall: Rich in nuts, seeds, late-season fruits, and an array of wildflowers. Remember that wildlife relies on these resources too, so strike a balance in your harvesting practices.

Winter: While foraging opportunities may seem scarce, winter provides unique finds like evergreen needles and leaves for tea or certain roots. In our climate pines, magnolias aund yaupon can be harvested all year.

FORAGING
ETHICALLY

Avoid foraging in protected areas, and always ask for permission if you're on private land. Harvest responsibly, leaving enough for the ecosystem to thrive and for other foragers to enjoy nature's gifts.

Familiarize yourself with the diverse plant species in your area. Invest in field guides, attend local workshops, or connect with experienced foragers who can share their knowledge. Learning to identify plants accurately is crucial for a safe and enjoyable foraging experience.

Foraging doesn't occur in isolation; it's a shared space with various creatures. Be conscious of their habitats and avoid disrupting ecosystems. Some plants serve as crucial food sources for wildlife, so leave ample resources for them to thrive.

Not all plants are safe to eat, and misidentification can have serious consequences. Cross-reference multiple sources, attend guided foraging walks, and start with easily identifiable species. If in doubt, it's best to err on the side of caution.

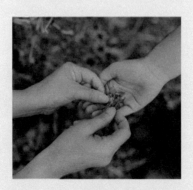

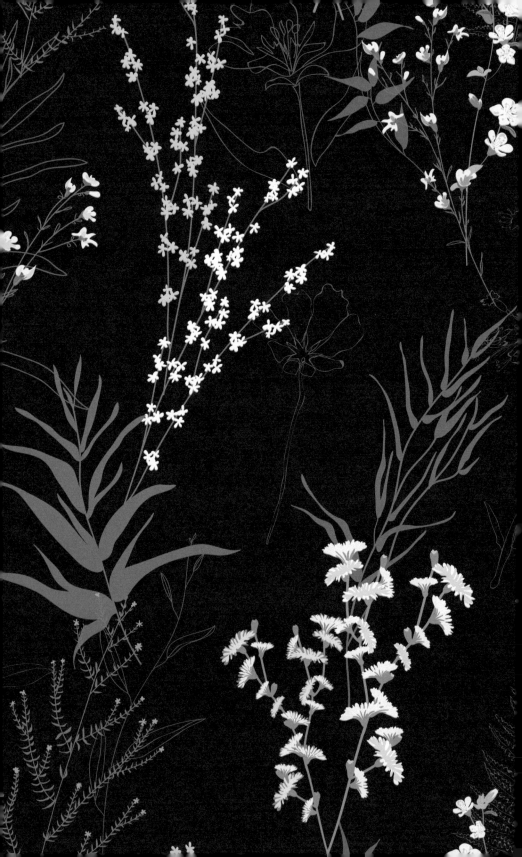

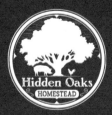

Happy Foraging!

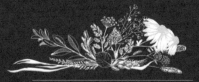

WHERE THE WILD THINGS GROW
APOTHECARY

Made in the USA
Columbia, SC
15 June 2024

37035811R00062